Handbook of
Cardiac Care

Handbook of Cardiac Care

K P Ball
J Fleming
T J Fowler
I James
G Maidment
C Ward

Published, in association with
Hastings Hilton Publishers Limited,
by

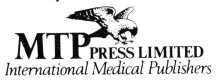

MTP PRESS LIMITED
International Medical Publishers

Published, in association with
Hastings Hilton Publishers Limited,
London,

by

MTP Press Limited
International Medical Publishers
Falcon House
Lancaster, England

Copyright © 1981 Update Books Ltd

First published 1981 as *The Heart Patient*

ISBN 0-85200-460-5

Printed in Great Britain

Contents

Contributors

K P Ball, MD, FRCP
Senior Lecturer in Preventive Medicine and Cardiology,
Middlesex Hospital Medical School, London

J Fleming MD, FRCP
Consultant Physician, Cardiothoracic Unit,
Northern General Hospital, Sheffield

T J Fowler, DM, FRCP
Consultant Neurologist for the South East Thames Region

Ian James, MB, PhD, FRCP
Senior Lecturer in Clinical Pharmacology,
Academic Departments of Medicine and Pharmacology,
Royal Free Hospital Medical School, London

Geoffrey Maidment, MB, MRCP
Senior Registrar, Norfolk & Norwich Hospital,
St Stephen's Road, Norwich

C Ward, MD, MRCP
Consultant Cardiologist at the
Regional Cardiothoracic Centre,
Wythenshawe Hospital,
Southmoor Road, Manchester

1
Is Heart Disease Preventable?

K. P. BALL

Great progress has been made in recent years in the treatment of heart disease as a result of the study of individual patients. It is a paradox that these advances have not prevented a steady increase in cardiovascular mortality, which now accounts for over half the deaths of middle-aged men and more than a quarter of those among middle-aged women. Most heart attacks and strokes occur suddenly in the apparently fit.

Prediction can therefore come only from the study of healthy people in the community in order to obtain clues for prevention. Fortunately this epidemiological approach is already showing great promise and has done much to indicate how heart disease might be prevented.

THE SIZE OF THE PROBLEM

Cardiovascular disease is the cause of 52% of the deaths of men aged 45 to 54 years, and 41% of those aged 35 to 44 years. It kills men during their most productive years and in women of these ages it is exceeded only by deaths from cancer (Figure 1.1).

Between 1950 and 1970, deaths from coronary heart disease (CHD) increased steadily, particularly in men, and also in women under the age of 45. In recent years there has been a tendency for this curve to flatten and it may be starting to fall, as has occurred already in the United States. Even if there is no further increase, the toll of preventable cardiovascular deaths is enormous.

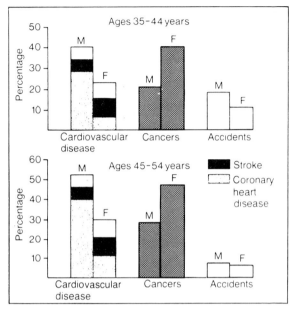

Figure 1.1   Causes of death in men and women aged 45 to 54 years and 35 to 44 years, in England and Wales, 1973. (From *Journal of the Royal College of Physicians,* 1976.)

INCIDENCE OF CARDIOVASCULAR DISEASE IN GENERAL PRACTICE

The average general practitioner with 2,500 patients on his list will see about seven deaths from coronary heart disease each year of which two may affect patients under the age of 65. Since one in five men will develop a heart attack before retirement, he will have about 100 such men on his list. In addition, there will be approximately four fatal strokes and one or two patients with lung cancer. However, the relative incidence of such conditions will depend very much on where he lives. Middle-class practices in the South of England have fewer patients with cardiovascular disease than do working class practices in the North, Ulster or Wales (Figure 1.2).

Wherever his practice is the general practitioner will find that a heart attack is the single commonest cause of death. Two-thirds are sudden and take place in the home, at work or during leisure. In

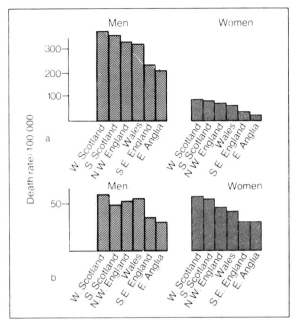

Figure 1.2 Observed death rates per 100,000 (averaged over 1969–77) in six regions in the UK, for a) coronary heart disease (ICD 410–414), and b) cerebrovascular disease (ICD 430–438). (From Fulton et al., *British Heart Journal,* 1978.)

about a quarter of all patients sudden death is the first manifestation of coronary heart disease, and the patient may perish unaware that he had anything wrong with his heart.

GENES VERSUS ENVIRONMENT IN CHD

Although a positive family history is more frequent among patients with CHD, man's environment is certainly much more important than his genes. Familial hyperlipidemia occurs in only one out of 250 of the population and can therefore not account for the large majority of cases.

The evidence for an environmental cause is as follows.

(1) *The wide variation in the incidence of CHD between different countries* (Figure 1.3). Scotland and Finland have

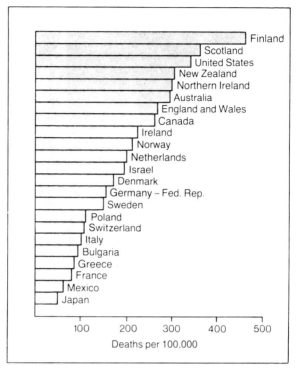

Figure 1.3   Mortality (deaths per 100,000) due to coronary heart disease in males aged 45 to 54 years, in 1971. (From *World Health Statistics Annual,* WHO, 1974.)

the highest incidence of CHD in the world, and England and Wales are only a little lower down the list. By contrast, the incidence of coronary heart disease in middle-aged Japanese men is less than one-tenth of that in Finland.

(2) *The experience of migrants moving from low- to high-risk countries.* Despite the low incidence of CHD in Japan, it is considerably higher in those Japanese who migrate to Hawaii, and second generation Japanese who have moved to California tend to resemble native Americans in their susceptibility to CHD (Figure 1.4). It is interesting that in those Japanese families which retain the traditional way of life there is no increased risk of CHD.

(3) *The steep rise in the incidence of CHD in many countries in*

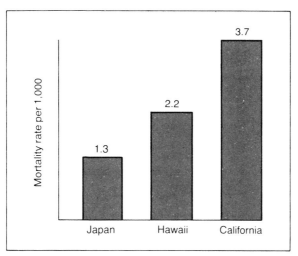

Figure 1.4 Average annual mortality rate for CHD per 1,000 for Japanese men aged 50 to 64, in their native country, Hawaii and California

recent years. This has been particularly marked among younger men where death rates due to CHD in England and Wales doubled between 1950 and 1970 (Figure 1.5).

(4) *The fall in deaths from CHD in wartime.*

(5) *Experimental evidence that rhesus monkeys develop arterial lesions similar to human atherosclerosis when put on Western type diets.*

It is clear that CHD is due mainly to the way we live and work. In recent years it has been possible to identify those factors, mainly behavioral, which lead to so many unnecessary deaths. CHD is the most important preventable disease in developed countries, but too little effort is made to take preventive steps at an early stage.

RISK FACTORS IN CHD

It is widely recognized that the main risk factors for CHD are cigarette smoking, raised serum cholesterol levels due mainly to diet, and high blood pressure. The risk is cumulative when more than one factor is present (Figure 1.6). Age, sex and family history

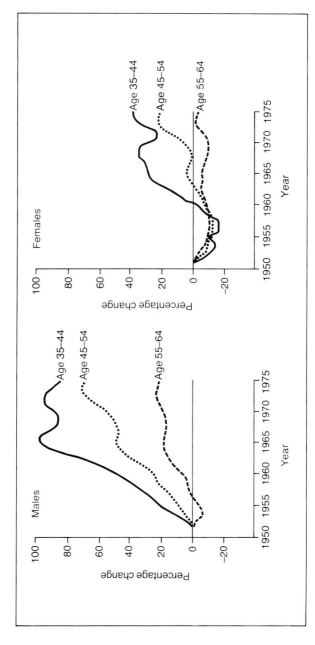

Figure 1.5 Percentage change in the death rates of males and females from coronary heart disease in England and Wales (1950–1975)

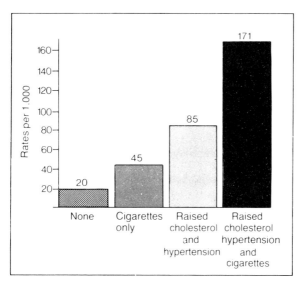

Figure 1.6 Additive effect of cigarettes, raised cholesterol and hypertension on the incidence of a first major coronary event. (From Inter Society Commission for Heart Diseases Resources, *Circulation*, 1970.)

are important risk indicators but clearly cannot be influenced. Diabetes, lack of exercise and excessive mental stress probably contribute to the development of CHD in some patients. Obesity, raised serum uric acid levels and soft water consumption are other, less clearly defined, associated factors.

1. Smoking

Each year above 40,000 men and women under the age of 65 in the UK die from CHD and about a quarter of those deaths are thought to be caused by cigarette smoking. For men under the age of 45 the risk is particularly great; those who smoke 25 or more cigarettes a day have a 10 to 15 fold increased risk of death (Figure 1.7), although the actual number of excess deaths from smoking is much greater over the age of 45, since coronary mortality rises rapidly with age. The marked increase of deaths from CHD between 1950 and 1970, especially among younger men, parallels the increase of cigarette smoking 25 years earlier (Figure 1.8). In younger women

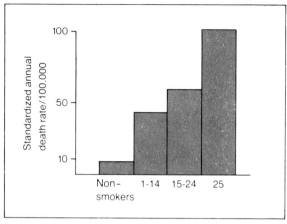

Figure 1.7   Annual mortality rate from coronary heart disease in men under 45 years of age. (Redrawn from Doll and Peto, 1976.)

an increase of CHD mortality occurred in England and Wales after 1960, perhaps related to increased cigarette smoking and the use of the contraceptive pill (Figure 1.5).

A much greater severity of atherosclerosis has been found in the coronary, peripheral and cerebral arteries at necropsy in smokers than in non-smokers.

Mechanisms

The two most important constituents of tobacco smoke which are thought to affect the heart are nicotine and carbon monoxide (Figure 1.9). The amount of nicotine absorbed from a cigarette varies from less than 0.3 mg to about 3.0 mg. The precise amount absorbed varies from about 5% for the non-inhaler to almost 100% for the deep inhaler. The heavy smoker who inhales may absorb 50 to 100 mg of nicotine daily. The main action of nicotine is to stimulate catecholamine production and its effects are therefore similar to those resulting from sympathetic overactivity. There is a rise in the pulse rate, blood pressure and cardiac output, with an increase in the force of myocardial contraction resulting in greater myocardial oxygen requirement. Smoking also causes increase in platelet stickiness and aggregation and has been found to inhibit fibrinolysis.

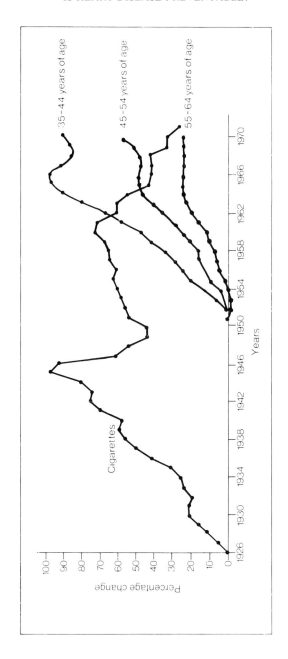

Figure 1.8 Percentage change in manufactured cigarette consumption in the UK (1926–1971) and in death rates for men from coronary heart disease in England and Wales in three age-groups (1950–1971)

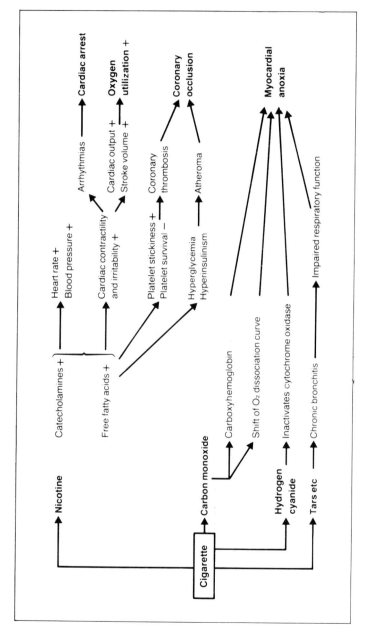

Figure 1.9 Some suggested mechanisms showing the association between cigarette smoking and coronary heart disease

Carbon monoxide

Cigarette smoke contains between 2.7 and 6% of carbon monoxide (CO) and when inhaled and diluted with air it contains about 400 parts per million, which is eight times greater than the maximum permitted level in industry. The affinity of hemoglobin for CO is about 200 times greater than that for oxygen which is therefore easily displaced. Carboxyhemoglobin (COHb) levels of up to 15 or 20% may be found in heavy smokers. CO shifts the oxygen dissociation curve to the left and thus impairs the release of oxygen to the tissues. In normal people, moderate COHb levels are followed by an increase in coronary blood flow, but when the coronary arteries are narrowed by atheroma, myocardial hypoxia may result.

CO therefore reduces the amount of oxygen available to the myocardium at a time when the work of the heart has been increased by the absorption of nicotine.

Does stopping help? Stopping smoking effectively reduces the risk of heart attack and is one of the most important preventive measures. In the Doll and Peto study the incidence of fatal coronary attacks was halved within five years in those aged under

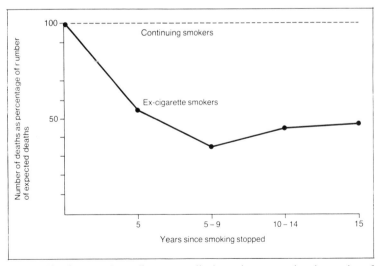

Figure 1.10 Coronary heart disease mortality in ex-cigarette smokers by number of years stopped smoking compared with mortality in continuing smokers. Men aged 30 to 54 years. (Redrawn from Doll and Peto, 1976.)

55 who stopped smoking (Doll and Peto, 1976) (Figure 1.10). Those who stopped after an infarct also halved their risk of relapse whether fatal or non-fatal. Helping patients to stop is probably the doctor's most effective action.

2. Diet and raised serum cholesterol levels

Many studies in different parts of the world have shown a clear correlation between raised serum cholesterol level and the risk of CHD. A man with a serum cholesterol level about 7.75 mmol/l (300 mg/100 ml) has more than three times the risk of a heart attack compared with the man whose cholesterol is less than 5.8 mmol/l (225 mg/100 ml) (Figure 1.11). Although normal levels of serum cholesterol for this country are often given as 3.6 mmol/l to 7.75 mmol/l (140 mg/100 ml to 300 mg/100 ml) this range cannot be considered normal in the sense of being healthy. In countries where the normal serum cholesterol levels are below 4.65 mmol/l (180 mg/100 ml), coronary heart disease is very rare despite the presence of other risk factors such as hypertension and cigarette smoking.

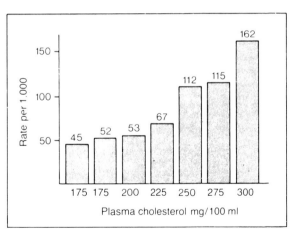

Figure 1.11 Plasma cholesterol and first major coronary events (including non-fatal myocardial infarction, fatal myocardial infarction and sudden death caused by coronary heart disease). Ten-year rates per 1,000 men aged 30 to 59 years at entry. (From Shaper, 1977, and the Editor of *Medicine,* with permission.)

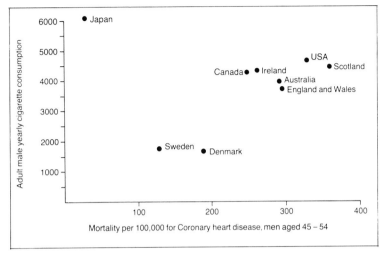

Figure 1.12 Mortality rate per 100,000 for coronary heart disease in men aged 45 to 54 and annual cigarette consumption

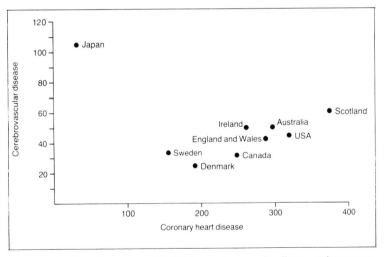

Figure 1.13 Mortality rate per 100,000 for cerebrovascular disease and coronary heart disease in men aged 45 to 54 in nine countries

Japan is an industrial country where smoking is heavy, hypertension common and CHD rare. In all countries except for Japan there is a good correlation between death rate from CHD and from

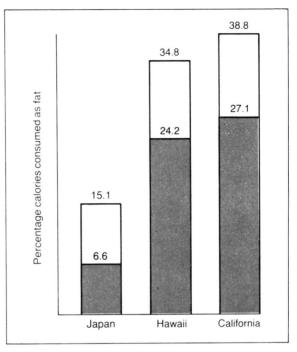

Figure 1.14   Percentage of calories consumed as total fat in Japanese men aged 45 to 69. The white area shows the percentage saturated fat. (From Kato *et al.*, 1973.)

either mean adult cigarette consumption (Figure 1.12) or death rate from strokes (Figure 1.13). A clear difference between the USA and Japan, related to their food pattern, is shown in their plasma cholesterol levels. Japanese migrants to Hawaii or California consume much more fat, a higher proportion of which is saturated (Figure 1.14). Likewise their consumption of carbohydrate, especially unrefined carbohydrate, falls (Figure 1.15). For a similar comparison of UK and Japanese diets see Table 1.1.

The relationship of dietary fats to CHD has been debated for many years. The matter has been reviewed by 20 national committees in 10 different countries. Each has recommended a reduction in the consumption of saturated fat either by the population as a whole or by those found on screening to be at high risk (Table 1.2). Nearly all advised a partial substitution of polyun-

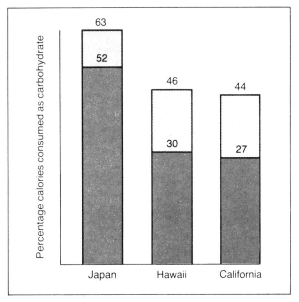

Figure 1.15 Percentage of calories consumed as total carbohydrate in Japanese men aged 45 to 69. The green coloured area shows the percentage complex carbohydrate. (From Kata *et al.*, 1973.)

saturated for saturated fat, and a reduction of dietary cholesterol. Many thought there should be an increased consumption of unrefined carbohydrate and that sugar intake should be reduced.

Table 1.1   Comparison of UK and Japanese diet. (From *Food Consumption Statistics*, OECD, 1973)

	g/person/day	
	UK	*Japan*
Dairy produce (not butter)	441	79
Meat	206	60
Sugar, sweets	136	74
Potatoes, etc	277	67
Cereals	198	348
Vegetables	169	372
Fish	23	94

Table 1.2   Recommendations of 20 committees from 10
countries on food and coronary heart disease

	General population
Reduction of saturated fats	20
Partial substitution with polyunsaturated fats	18
Reduction of dietary cholesterol	18
Reduction of sugar	14
. Labelling of fat content of food	13

Saturated fat

The main source of saturated fat is dairy produce, although meat
and meat products, hydrogenated vegetable and marine oils make a
substantial contribution. Nearly half our fat intake is of dairy
origin and half of this comes from butter and cream. It is recommended that there should be a reduction in the consumption of
fats, particularly saturated fats of animal and vegetable origin.

Polyunsaturated fat

In countries where most of the fat taken is polyunsaturated (corn
oil, soya bean oil, sunflower seed oil, etc.) or is monounsaturated
(olive oil), serum cholesterol levels are usually low and CHD
uncommon. The use of polyunsaturated fats helps to lower serum
cholesterol levels and to counteract the opposing effect of saturated
fat. In addition they help to reduce platelet stickiness and thrombus
formation. Many authorities have recommended a diet which
derives 30 to 35% of its calories from fat; one-third each from
saturated, monounsaturated and polyunsaturated fat. Most
patients find such diets acceptable and soon grow accustomed to
cutting down on their previous high intake of saturated fat, refined
carbohydrates and excess calories. There is no evidence that polyunsaturated fats taken in such amounts have any harmful effect.
There is in fact growing evidence that diets high in saturated fat
may actually increase the risk of carcinoma of the breast, colon and
pancreas.

Cholesterol

Dietary cholesterol contributes about 25 to 30% to the serum cholesterol. Most authorities recommend a reduction to about 300 mg a day. Since an egg contains about 250 mg, and meat and milk products also contain cholesterol, it is advisable to limit the number of eggs to three a week, especially for those otherwise at high risk.

The implications of these facts led The Royal College of Physicians and the British Cardiac Society Committee to advise:

(1) Eat less meat and fewer egg yolks, eat more poultry and fish. Choose lean meat and remove visible fat from meat. Broil rather than fry.
(2) Use butter sparingly; preferably use a soft margarine high in polyunsaturated fats. In general, avoid cream.
(3) Use oils rich in polyunsaturated fats for cooking, e.g. corn oil, sunflower oil, safflower oil. Avoid hard margarines or lard. Oils labelled merely 'vegetable oil' may contain a large amount of saturated fat and very little polyunsaturated fat and should be avoided.
(4) Eat more vegetables and fruit of all kinds.

3. Hypertension

High blood pressure contributes to much cardiovascular disease and death. It is a potent cause of CHD and causes more deaths from heart attacks and heart failure than from strokes. A man aged 35 with a blood pressure of 160/100 mmHg – a level which many would not consider unduly serious – has his expectation of life reduced by an average of $16\frac{1}{2}$ years. Compared with a man whose blood pressure is 120/80, who can expect to live to $76\frac{1}{2}$ years, he can expect to survive only until age 60. The risk of even mildly elevated blood pressure has been repeatedly confirmed. However, this does not mean that every person with a blood pressure of 160/100 mmHg should immediately be put on drugs.

Mild degrees of hypertension being so common in the UK lead to many more cases of CHD than those few with marked hypertension. Fortunately the incidence of fatal strokes, both in

UK and America, has been falling for many years, probably due to the combined effect of lower salt consumption with wide use of food refrigeration and also, although probably to a lesser extent, to drug treatment. This reduction of hypertensive disease may be one cause of the fall in coronary mortality in the USA and Australia, and a flattening out in the UK. Yet in Japan, with the highest stroke mortality in the world, CHD is uncommon.

Incidence of raised blood pressure in general practice

It has been found that 40% of men aged 45 to 64 have a diastolic blood pressure of 90 mmHg or more, 16%, 100 mmHg or more, and 3%, 115 mmHg or more. This means that for middle-aged men alone an average general practitioner is likely to have about 100 with a diastolic pressure above 90 mmHg, 50 above 100 mmHg and about 10 above 115 mmHg. It has been found that usually only about half of the patients with a raised blood pressure have been recognized previously, and only half of these have been receiving treatment of which in only a half again was the treatment effective.

The risks of raised blood pressure

A single blood pressure reading is a potent predictor of the risk of CHD, and the first reading of systolic blood pressure seems to be as clear a predictor as is the diastolic blood pressure or repeated blood pressure readings. The risk of CHD increases continuously with no evident threshold (Figure 1.16). The patient with a very high blood pressure faces a particularly great risk of stroke or left ventricular failure. However, it is mild hypertension which contributes most to the occurrence of CHD, because it is so much more prevalent than the severe form. From the community point of view, the greater part of this risk relates to those with a diastolic blood pressure of below 100 mmHg.

Management

How should I manage a 35-year-old man with a blood pressure of 160/100 mmHg? In the first place he should not be given a drug to lower his blood pressure – at least not until other measures have

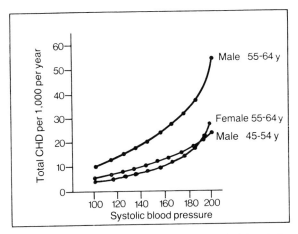

Figure 1.16   CHD incidence (averaged over a 16-year period) in relation to blood pressure at initial examination. (From *Journal of the Royal College of Physicians*, 1976.)

been tried. His main risk is of developing a coronary attack. The risk of a stroke is much less, at least for several years. Giving the patient drug treatment from the start is likely to absolve him from first taking responsibility for changes in his life style which he may find unpleasant. A mild hypertensive who stops smoking, reduces dietary fats and total calories, cuts down his salt intake and takes regular physical exercise is likely to improve his outlook much more than if he merely takes a drug to lower his blood pressure. He will certainly feel much better and avoid any side-effects. These measures often lead to a fall in blood pressure and the need for drugs disappears. A careful follow-up is required every 6 to 12 months to check blood pressure and other habits, and should the blood pressure not respond to these measures, drug treatment will, of course, be needed.

4. Diabetes

In the West, arterial disease is the most important cause of disability and death due to diabetes, and the outlook of the diabetic following a heart attack is poor. A recent study showed that half the diabetic patients admitted to hospital for a myocardial

Table 1.3 Mortality rates (per cent) from arterial and reno-
vascular disease among American and Japanese diabetics

	USA	Japan
Coronary	53.3	6.5
Cerebral	12.4	11.1
Gangrene	1.3	0.3
Renovascular	9.2	19.3

Table 1.4 Calorie distribution in American and Japanese
diabetic diets

	USA	Japan
	(per cent)	
Carbohydrate	40	60
Protein	15	15
Fat	45	25

infarction were dead by one year. Yet there is little evidence that
current methods of treatment have reduced the toll of diabetic
atherosclerosis. This is only the case in Western cultures since in
diabetic populations in Africa and Asia CHD rarely occurs (Table
1.3). For many years the traditional diabetic diets in the UK and
USA have been low in carbohydrate and hence relatively high in
fat. It has been found that only 8 or 9% of diabetic clinics in the
UK advised fat restriction for their patients.

Diabetic diets in the UK and USA have been low in carbohydrate
and consequently high in fat, and it is likely that such diets may
have increased the risk of arterial disease (Table 1.4).

Recently it has been shown that diabetic control is better
achieved by giving high carbohydrate diets, especially when given
unrefined and uncooked. Certain specific unabsorbable carbohydrate such as guars and pectins have been shown to improve
diabetic control and to lower plasma cholesterol levels. Present
methods of treatment do not reduce the risk of arterial disease in
diabetics. It is therefore particularly important to make sure that
the diabetic does not smoke, that his hypertension is controlled,
and that his exercise is adequate. Most important of all, his blood
lipids must be examined, his diet must be high in carbohydrate and
low in fat, and the saturated fat in the diet must be partially
replaced with polyunsaturated fats. By these means diabetic arterial
complications could probably be considerably reduced.

5. Physical activity

There is growing evidence that lack of exercise contributes to the development of coronary heart disease and may be an important reason why men of social class V (unskilled workers) now exceed professional men in their risk of fatal CHD. The forklift truck, the mechanical digger and the conveyor belt have reduced the need for physical effort in many working men. Housewives rarely scrub or polish floors, hang out heavy washing or even turn mattresses. Labour saving has become a major objective for which we may have to pay a heavy price. Although heavy exercise in Finnish lumber jacks does not protect them in the presence of other strong risk factors, many studies have shown that those undertaking vigorous exercise have a reduced risk of CHD. Today physical activity must be found more in leisure than at work. The study of middle-aged Civil Servants showed that those undertaking vigorous exercise such as cycling and swimming or heavy gardening have about one-third the incidence of CHD compared with those who did not.

Regular vigorous exercise improves cardiopulmonary function and exercise tolerance and increases fibrinolytic activity. In smokers it speeds the elimination of carbon monoxide. All forms of rhythmic dynamic exercise are beneficial if energetic, such as brisk walking, jogging, swimming or cycling. Motivating the middle-aged to exercise would be encouraged by provision of better facilities including more swimming baths and cycle lanes.

After a coronary heart attack early return to work and former leisure activities is recognized as the best form of rehabilittion for most patients. The man who loses weight, stops smoking and walks to work after his coronary attack usually feels better than he did before it.

6. Obesity

Although obesity is associated with an increased risk of death from CHD, by itself it is probably not a major cause. Those who are overweight yet are not diabetic, hypertensive or physically inert and whose blood lipids and uric acid levels are normal are no more likely to succumb to heart attacks than their thinner brothers or sisters. Obesity's bad reputation seems to rest on its frequent association with these other factors rather than to the presence of surplus adipose tissue. Those with primary obesity are less at risk than those who put on weight after the age of 25.

However, men who are 20% or more overweight have a 35% excess mortality from CHD, and control of obesity is an important way of helping to reduce raised blood pressure and plasma cholesterol and to control diabetes. Obesity should therefore be considered a likely indicator of other risk factors which should be carefully investigated and controlled.

7. Stress

In recent years careful studies have helped to define the possible role of stress as a risk factor in CHD. Engineers use the term 'stress' for the force exerted on the body and 'strain' for the deformity produced. The term stress is here considered to mean the individual's adverse reaction to environmental or endogenous stimuli.

Acute manifestations

Acute mental stress can precipitate angina pectoris, left ventricular failure, myocardial infarction, arrhythmias and sudden death, probably due to the effects of excess catecholamine secretion in patients who already have diseased coronary arteries. Sudden fright may also lead to vagal stimulation with bradycardia or even cardiac arrest. Potentially lethal arrhythmias have been recorded in coronary care units at the time of cardiac arrest in another patient. It would be surprising if the emergency ambulance journey did not sometimes have a similar effect. Sudden death is usually caused by ventricular fibrillation, a rhythm disturbance which can be precipitated by emotional shock. Precipitation of angina or left ventricular failure by anger or excitement is well known, as when watching horseracing or football on television.

Life changes

Stressful events may precede coronary attacks. Such events as the death of a spouse, divorce, business problems or loss of a job have been found to be more frequent in the months before a coronary attack than in control populations. A marked increase in death rates of both widows and widowers has been found within one year of their bereavement, particularly from CHD.

ECG changes

Emotional stress such as that produced by public speaking or car driving can cause ventricular ectopic beats and ST depression in those with apparently healthy hearts, but these changes are more marked in those with CHD.

Although the assessment of mental tension can be difficult there seems little doubt that mental stress, whether acute or long-standing, can be an important factor in the development of coronary heart attacks. The physician must learn to recognise warning symptoms especially in those with other risk factors such as hypertension and cigarette smoking.

Personality type

There is some evidence that certain behavior patterns are more frequent in coronary prone patients. Friedman and Rosenman have described the Type A personality as one involving 'intense striving for achievement, competitiveness, aggressiveness, pressure for vocational productivity, excessive sense of time urgency, impatience and restlessness'. Such patients are said to have a higher risk of CHD, even when such factors as cigarette smoking are taken into account.

Management of stress

A good doctor will become aware of the patient who is steering his ship towards the rocks. Examples are the middle-aged man whose drive and ambition have brought too rapid promotion, his business success often contrasting with discord at home; or the heavy smoking woman attempting to run both a career and a home, known to have mild hypertension and taking the contraceptive pill; or the self-employed artisan who knows no set working hours and who has not taken his family on holiday for years. These are the people who need unhurried counselling, yet are often too occupied to find the time or fail to recognize the need. Fear of a coronary attack is often present among such people who need help to get off their self-imposed treadmills or at least to slow them down.

The fear of death often accompanies the onset of an acute coronary attack and the events which follow often aggravate rather than relieve this stress. The rush to hospital by ambulance, the arrival in a coronary care unit surrounded by unfamiliar instruments can accentuate anxiety. Although an opiate combined with the reassuring efficiency of the unit may give temporary relief, the patient soon starts to worry about his mortgage, the business, his children and his possible return to work. A reassuring attitude by the staff is not only humane but may help to reduce catecholamine secretion and be directly therapeutic. A full discussion of all those factors thought to have brought on the attack should be carried out with both patient and spouse before leaving hospital and later with the general practitioner before returning to work.

8. Congenital heart disease

In about 1 to 4% of babies born with heart defects, maternal rubella may be the cause. Every year 1 in 200 babies is born with a congenital rubella syndrome and many such have congenital heart defects. Since this form of congenital heart disease is preventable it is essential to make sure that all girls and women of child-bearing age are protected. The campaign to vaccinate girls aged 11 to 14 should help to reduce the number of babies with the rubella syndrome in future. Women who think they have had German measles have only a 50% chance of being right. Certainty can come only from testing. All women not vaccinated should be tested and those found to be non-immune should be vaccinated. This is particularly important for nurses of both sexes in obstetrics units since development of rubella could be a hazard to mothers attending antenatal clinics.

9. Uric acid

The serum uric acid level varies with age, sex, weight, social class and alcohol intake. Some hold that uric acid is an independent risk factor for coronary heart disease but others have shown that the association of uric acid and CHD is mediated through other factors. Hyperuricemic subjects tend to be more obese and have a higher prevalence of glucose intolerance and raised packed cell volume. Hypertriglyceridemia is associated with raised serum uric acid levels and occurs in more than 80% of patients with gout. About one-third of untreated hypertensive patients are hyperuricemic. Furthermore, treatment with thiazide diuretics and adrenergic blocking agents may cause hyperuricemia.

In the Framingham study a significant association was noted in some age groups between serum uric acid and the incidence of CHD. It was also found the ECG changes suggesting CHD were more frequent in hyperuricemic patients. The mean uric acid levels of men who died from CHD and cardiovascular disease were found to be higher than in those who survived. However, this association did not persist after control for other risk factors and use of diuretics.

It was concluded that raised serum uric acid levels could be an independent risk factor for CHD in women but its association with ECG abnormalities and the incidence of CHD in men could be considered secondary to association with hypertension, obesity and the use of diuretics.

10. Oral contraceptives

In the large study by the Royal College of General Practitioners, cardiovascular deaths were increased five times in women taking oral contraceptives and ten times in those who had done so for five years or more. The excess was substantially greater than the death rate from complications of pregnancy in the controls and was double the death rate from accidents. A study of mortality trends in 21 countries suggested that an increase of deaths from all non-rheumatic heart diseases had occurred in women aged 15 to 44 since the introduction of oral contraceptives.

The risk is greater in women with other risk factors such as cigarette smoking, raised serum cholesterol levels, diabetes or hypertension. In older women the risk increases, especially in those who smoke cigarettes. Should such a woman wish to continue on the Pill she should certainly stop smoking. If unwilling or unable to do so she should be advised to change to an alternative method of contraception.

RHEUMATIC HEART DISEASE

The dramatic fall in the prevalence of rheumatic heart disease in this country is a happy reminder than one type of cardiovascular disease can be controlled, and there is no reason why coronary and hypertensive heart disease should not follow the same pattern. Table 1.5 shows the virtual disappearance of rheumatic heart disease as a problem in general practice, mainly due to improved social conditions and the use of antibiotics.

Unfortunately rheumatic fever and carditis remain a major problem in many tropical countries in association with strepto-coccal infection and malnutrition, and there is an increased incidence in migrants from these countries.

Table 1.5   Patients consulting (aged 45 to 64) per 1,000 on practitioners' lists. (From Second National General Practice Morbidity Survey, 1970–71)

Diagnosis	Men	Women
Coronary heart disease	33	13
Hypertension, etc	31	44
Cerebrovascular disease	6.2	3.9
Peripheral arterial disease, other 'arteriosclerosis', etc	8.1	5.1
Rheumatic fever and heart disease	1.5	3.3

THE FUTURE

Mortality rates for middle-aged men (55 to 64 years of age) started to fall in about the year 1900, but in the last 30 years have remained almost static. Any further decline has been cancelled by the increase of coronary heart disease and lung cancer, both preventable conditions. Between them they cause 43,000 deaths a year in men of working age (35 to 64 years of age) in England and Wales, amounting to 46% of all deaths in this age-group.

We know many of the factors which lead to CHD. It is recognized that cigarette smoking and lack of physical exercise can be important factors and recommended that the amount of fat in the diet, especially saturated fat from both animal and plant sources, should be reduced. On some levels very little has been done. Millions of pounds are spent in informing us that certain cigarettes are 'the best money can buy', or that we should drink a 'pint of milk a day'.

We know that man's environment is the main cause of cardio-vascular disease and that it surrounds him from the day he is born. Fetal blood vessels can be damaged by maternal smoking. The antigenic effects of cow's milk and weaning onto a diet rich in saturated fats, refined carbohydrates and salt may add further insults. The child today naturally considers the food he is given to be normal, although it is far removed from the natural diet on which man has evolved. At school he learns to smoke, and on leaving school his life of physical inactivity often starts. If he becomes a 'manual labourer' he finds that modern technology has provided him with a sedentary job. His wife's housework is now almost devoid of physical activity since she no longer scrubs the clothes, turns the mattresses or polishes the floors. The 'convenience' foods she gives her family leave her unaware of what they contain.

It is clear that the major reduction in deaths from CHD will not take place until, as a nation, we change our ways of eating,

Table 1.6   Changes in risk factors between fathers (1948–50) and sons (1971–75) at ages 35–39: Framingham offspring study

	Difference			
Systolic BP (mmHg)	− 6.0	(132.1	⟶	126.1)
Cigarette smoking (per cent)	− 35%	(74	⟶	39%)
Plasma cholesterol (mg/100 ml)	− 8.2	(213	⟶	204.5)

smoking and exercise. The seeds of CHD are sown in childhood and it is essential that healthy habits start here. It is as important for the general practitioner to advise his younger patients and their parents on these matters as on immunization.

Discovering the higher risk adult must also be his responsibility. A hemiplegic stroke occurring in a woman whose blood pressure has never been recorded, or a fatal coronary attack in an over-weight, heavy smoking man who has never been advised, both indicate substandard care.

One of the most encouraging developments in recent years has been the fall in mortality from CHD in the USA. Between 1969 and 1977 death rates fell by 19.5% in white men and 24% in white women. Rates have also been falling in Australia and Finland. In the USA there has been widespread health education on smoking, exercise and diet. That there have been changes in behavior over the last 30 years is supported by figures from the Framingham Offspring Study in which findings in parents were compared with those in their children some 25 years later (Table 1.6). At ages 35 to 39 the sons had a systolic blood pressure 6.0 mmHg lower, plasma cholesterol 8.2 mg lower and little more than half the percentage of cigarette smoking than their fathers at the same age.

In 1968 death rates from CHD for men aged 45 to 54 were 41% higher in the USA than in England and Wales. While UK rates have remained static, by 1977 US rates had fallen below UK rates. We cannot be sure that the health education campaigns conducted especially by the heart foundations and health departments in some countries, in contrast to others, have been the major cause of their improved health record; but it certainly suggests that their efforts may have been an important factor.

The current policy of waiting for proof which cannot be obtained, before action is taken on the prevention of coronary heart disease, will surely be strongly criticized by future genera-tions. Dietary modification following the consensus of international opinion, combined with a significant reduction in cigarette smoking and an encouragement for young and old alike to increase physical activity could bring a significant reduction in coronary mortality within 10 years. No other method is likely to achieve such results.

References

Doll, R. and Peto, R. (1976). *Br. Med. J.,* **2,** 1525
Food Consumption Statistics, OECD, 1973
Fulton, M., Adams, W., Lutz, W. and Oliver, M. F. (1978). *Br. Heart J.,* **40,** 563
Inter Society Commission for Heart Disease Resources, (1970). *Circulation,* **42,** A55
Journal of the Royal College of Physicians, (1976). 10, 1
Kato, *et al.* (1973). *Am. J. Epidemiol.,* **97,** 372
Shaper, G. (1977). *Medicine,* **26,** 1326

Further Reading

Auerback *et al.* (1965). *New Engl. J. Med.,* **273,** 775
Wilhelmsson, C., Vedin, J. A., Elmfeldt, D., Tibblin, G. and Wilhelmsen, L. (1975). *Lancet,* **i,** 415

2
Case Finding in General Practice

K. P. BALL

Many of the factors predisposing to cardiovascular disease are known. They are prevalent in the healthy, or at least in the symptom-free, population. Simple logic would suggest that their detection could lead to prevention. Many screening trials have been carried out, many high-risk patients detected and much advice and treatment has been given; yet screening remains one of the most controversial subjects in medicine.

Important questions remain unanswered. Can we modify the course of the disease detected? Detection of a condition we cannot influence is clearly but harmful interference. Does knowledge of risk induce unnecessary anxiety? This must depend on the degree of risk and the chance of modifying it. If advice is given will people take it? We know that poor compliance is common whether with advice on smoking, keeping to diets or taking pills. Yet should those who are prepared to change behavior not be given the chance?

Is mass screening cost effective? Should we not rather turn to the detection by the general practitioner of the 'at-risk' patient in the course of normal practice?

Clear distinction needs to be made between mass screening of a population for early disease, such as by mass X-ray or blood pressure measurement, and the detection of symptom-free, but high-risk individuals by the general practitioner in the course of his work. The Joint Working Party of The Royal College of Physicians and British Cardiac Society considered that 'the prevention of CHD in the community is predominantly the role of the general practitioner'. Indeed, he is in a far better position to influence his patients if he finds raised blood pressure, obesity or heavy smoking, than if these are discovered through an impersonal screening service. Discovering pulmonary tuberculosis on mass X-ray leads to referral of the patient for specialist treatment, which is usually beyond the scope of the general practitioner. Most coronary risk factors are easily detected but, by contrast, their modification often involves changes of behavior that can better be controlled by the advice and support of a general practitioner and his team.

The measures outlined in this chapter are those which the family doctor, with the help of his community nurse or health visitor, could take with a reasonable chance of reducing the incidence of coronary heart attacks and strokes in his patients. Such advice is not only relevant to the patient who is well but also to one who has already had a heart attack or stroke.

IDENTIFYING THE HIGH-RISK PATIENT

In any one year about 60% of patients consult their general practitioner and within five years nearly all are seen. Some practitioners also interview all new patients they take on their lists. This provides a good opportunity for the high-risk patient to be identified provided that the procedure can be fitted into the practice routine: a suitable record would include family history, occupation, smoking, exercise, blood pressure and weight. In this way most risk factors could be easily determined and a decision made as to which patients required a more detailed health examination.

It may not be possible to prove that such simple enquiry under-taken by the doctor or his health visitor or nurse reduces the incidence of disease in his practice, but it is likely to be reassuring to the patient to know that his doctor takes an interest in his life-style; advice from his doctor on specific points is probably the most effective type of health education.

Selective health examination

The initial short enquiry will detect certain patients who need fuller examination and more detailed advice. These will include:

(1) Those with a strong family history of sudden death, angina pectoris, stroke or hypertension, or where one member has had a heart attack, especially if under the age of 50.
(2) Those who have several risk factors, such as hypertension, smoking and obesity.

As a result, some people will be given special advice. A smoking patient will be advised to stop, and follow-up appointments will be arranged to give him support. A patient found to have symptomless hypertension may be advised to reduce weight, cut salt intake, stop smoking and increase exercise. The combination of cigarette smoking and the use of the contraceptive pill in women over the age of 35 needs particular attention. Reinforcement of advice should be given by suitable pamphlets, such as those produced by The Health Education Council. The doctor's advice on specific factors should be written down: it is too easy for the patient to forget advice when it involves his way of living!

The visiting nurse may wish to visit some high-risk families to discuss some of the problems and give dietary advice. She can explain that non-smoking parents are less likely to have children who smoke.

By enquiry and selective examination the doctor will discover those of his patients at highest risk from coronary heart disease and armed with this knowledge, he is then in a position to instigate preventive measures.

Further tests

In those patients found, by selective health examination, to be at greater risk of heart disease, it is advisable to take blood for lipid estimation. The patient with a plasma cholesterol of more than 300 mg/100 ml (7.75 mmol) has more than three times the risk of a coronary attack compared with one whose cholesterol is less than 200 mg/100 ml (5.2 mmol). Lipid estimation therefore helps greatly to increase prediction: recently it has been suggested that the ratio of HDL to LDL (or HDL to total cholesterol) gives the best prediction.

In trained hands an electrocardiogram can help to identify those at greatest risk. Well marked left axis deviation with flattening or inversion of T waves in the left chest leads is associated with a greater likelihood of a coronary attack. However, the main use of an ECG in general practice is in the assessment of hypertension and in helping to clarify the cause of chest pain. Recognition and interpretation of specific abnormalities need both experience and a good apparatus, since false positive and false negative findings occur frequently.

IS DETECTION IN GENERAL PRACTICE FEASIBLE?

Some practitioners may feel that the detection of high-risk patients unduly increases their work and that their main duty is to treat patients with symptoms. Others have found that with the help of the visiting nurse service it is possible to introduce a simple scheme of surveillance. An age–sex register enables the doctor to ensure that all patients in a specific age group are screened, for example men between 40 and 60 years of age. Such a procedure should involve the doctor in limited extra work and, although he would need to give any necessary advice, only those with unfavourable features would require a more detailed examination.

RESULTS OF GENERAL PRACTITIONER CASE-FINDING

Russell *et al.* (1979) found that of patients advised to stop smoking by their practitioners during a routine visit to the surgery, and who were given leaflets and warned that they would be followed up, 5.1% were still not smoking after a year. In contrast only 0.3% given no advice managed to stop. The result suggested that any general practitioner who adopted this simple routine could expect about 25 long-term successes in one year, which could be of great significance for the prevention of heart and lung diseases.

The effect of routine blood pressure screening in general practice is less certain. In a controlled trial, conducted in south-east London

(D'Souza *et al.* 1976), to evaluate the results of screening (especially for hypertension), no significant benefit was found for the screened group after five years. Furthermore, it was noted that over 95% of the new hypertensives discovered by screening had visited their general practitioner at some time during this period. In another study from Glasgow (Barber *et al.* 1979) it was concluded that a population could be examined routinely through normal contact with the family doctor, which could provide a convenient, acceptable and effective means of detecting and reducing raised blood pressure. Tudor Hart believes that the general practitioner should know the blood pressure of every man and woman between the ages of 35 and 64 in his practice, and has shown that this is feasible and can be done.

The finding of a raised blood pressure does not mean that antihypertensive drugs should be immediately prescribed. However, it does identify the patient at significantly greater risk of heart disease. It can be just as important to advise him about smoking, exercise and diet – particularly where raised serum cholesterol levels are found – as to put him on drugs. If after three months his blood pressure remains raised, then a thiazide diuretic and/or a beta-blocking drug should be prescribed.

Even the occasional finding of severe symptomless hypertension, for example 200/120 mmHg or higher, should make regular blood pressure estimation worthwhile, since the risk of stroke is much reduced by treatment. Dr Coope, a general practitioner from Macclesfield, records finding a patient with a diastolic blood pressure of 170 mmHg, who had attended for ear syringing! Every practice may well have such a patient.

WHO SHOULD DO THE WORK?

Much of the specialist and technical work of doctors, such as cardiac resuscitation and renal dialysis, is today being undertaken by nurses. It is clear that a trained nurse can also do much of the case finding, examination and health education in general practice. She can measure the blood pressure and, if necessary, record an electrocardiogram and take blood. The regulation that sometimes prevents nurses from taking blood is absurd. Nurses are likely to take more interest in such regular tests than doctors who can then concentrate on diagnosis and treatment.

CONCLUSIONS

Between the extremes of those who advocate mass population screening and those who feel their responsibility is only for symptomatic patients, there seems to be a growing recognition of a middle course: the development of anticipatory care. The identification of patients at risk from preventable conditions is becoming increasingly recognized as an important element in good medical practice.

However, the discovery of predictors of cardiovascular disease in symptom-free adults may yet be too late. Many men have been free from symptoms right up to their sudden death, after which widespread disease of all their coronary arteries is found. Health education must start much earlier because the seeds of coronary disease are sown in childhood. In future we must strive to bring up children free from cigarette smoke, on nourishing diets which do not promote atherosclerosis and with an enjoyment of exercise that becomes a lifelong habit. Could we reach this ideal, cardiovascular disease might become as rare as pulmonary tuberculosis is today and the need for screening disappear.

References

Barber, J. H., Beevers, D. G., Fife, R., Hawthorne, V. M., McKenzie, H. M., Sinclair, R. G., Simpson, R. J., Stewart, G. M. and Williams, D. I. (1979). *Br. Med. J.,* **1**, 843

D'Souza, M. F., Swan, A. V. and Shannon, D. J. (1976). *Lancet,* **ii**, 1128

Russell, M. A. H., Wilson, C., Taylor, C. and Baker, C. D. (1979). *Br. Med. J.,* **2**, 231

3
The Unexpected Finding on Routine Examination

C. WARD and J. FLEMING

There are many situations in which an unexpected finding on routine examination suggests the possibility of underlying cardio-vascular disease, for example, during insurance or pre-employment examinations and at preschool medicals. Many of us occasionally receive detailed reports from private medical insurance schemes which some firms offer as a service to their employees. Further-more, an increasing number of patients are requesting a routine examination 'just to make sure...'.

The discovery of an abnormality under these circumstances in-evitably raises several questions.

(1) Is the unexpected finding due to disease or is it a normal variant?
(2) If it is abnormal, what action, if any, should be taken?

It is fair to say that almost any type of heart disease may occasionally be detected in an asymptomatic patient. Clearly it is impossible to include all the possibilities, and we shall concentrate on the more common unexpected findings. Although this concerns asymptomatic patients it is worth bearing in mind that a patient's claim to be symptom-free should not always be taken at face value. A patient with chronically progressive heart disease may have gradually limited his activities and come to accept as normal what is, in fact, a markedly restricted existence.

Unexpected abnormalities can, for convenience, be grouped under two headings: first, clinical examination and second, routine laboratory investigations.

ABNORMAL FINDINGS ON EXAMINATION

Hyperlipidemia

Preliminary inspection may provide evidence suggestive of hyper-lipidemia. Several cutaneous manifestations may be apparent, the commonest of which are arcus senilis and xanthelasma.

Arcus senilis

Arcus senilis (Figure 3.1) is a time-honoured pointer to degenera-tive arterial disease. This white ring at the periphery of the cornea consists of deposited cholesterol and is an abnormal finding in patients under the age of 45 years, signifying the probability of hypercholesterolemia. The incidence of coronary artery disease is high in such patients. Estimation of fasting serum lipids is worth-while, since the correction of any abnormality detected may prevent future trouble. With advancing years the significance of the

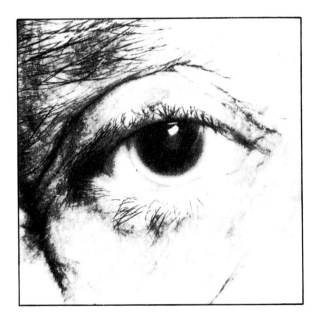

Figure 3.1   Xanthomata over the Achilles tendon

corneal arcus diminishes and it may be regarded as a normal finding in the elderly.

Xanthelasma

Xanthelasmata are small elevated yellowish lesions on the upper or lower eyelids containing cholesterol. It has been suggested that repeated minor trauma from rubbing the eyes causes extravasation of blood into the tissue and that if the cholesterol level is high, incomplete reabsorption results in the persistence of yellow plaques. The significance of xanthelasma is similar to that of the arcus senilis.

Other cutaneous clues

Other cutaneous manifestations of hyperlipidemia, although much less common, are more closely associated with abnormal lipid

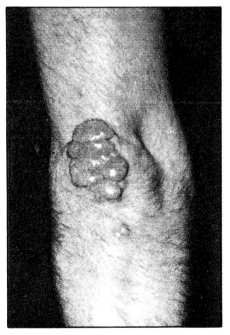

Figure 3.2   Tuberous xanthomata on the elbow

patterns. Tendon xanthomata are hard nodules on the knuckles and in the patellar and Achilles tendons and these nodules are pathognomonic of hypercholesterolemia. Tuberous xanthomata, subcutaneous nodules on the knees, elbows (Figure 3.2) and buttocks, are equally significant. The discovery of any of these manifestations of hyperlipidemia warrants assessment of plasma lipids. The justification for, and principles of, treatment are outlined later.

The pulse

Examination of the pulse may reveal evidence of an arrhythmia of which the patient is unaware but which can nevertheless indicate underlying heart disease requiring either investigation or treatment. In many cases electrocardiography is required to establish the precise nature of the arrhythmia and its significance.

An irregular pulse

Irregularity of the pulse is usually due to sinus arrhythmia, ectopic beats or atrial fibrillation.

Sinus arrhythmia. This is a normal cyclical variation in heart rate in which the pulse rate increases during inspiration (Figure 3.3). It is particularly common in children, in whom the irregularity may be striking.

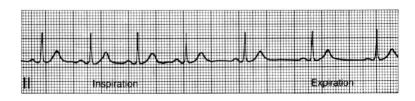

Figure 3.3   Sinus arrhythmia. During inspiration the heart rate is faster than during expiration

Ventricular ectopic beats. Ectopic beats may be appreciated by the patient as 'missed' beats although in many cases he is unaware of their presence. The typical finding is of irregularly occurring 'gaps' in the pulse followed by a beat of increased force (Figure 3.4). Ventricular ectopic beats are justifiably viewed with some suspicion because they often occur in serious heart disease and may initiate ventricular tachycardia or ventricular fibrillation. This, however, is not always so and it has been estimated that about 1% of healthy

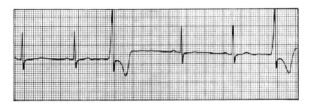

Figure 3.4   Unifocal ventricular ectopics. They are identical in appearance and therefore arise from the same ventricular focus

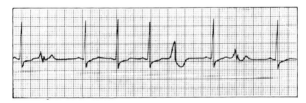

Figure 3.5   Multifocal ventricular ectopics. Since their shapes are so different they must arise from more than one focus in the ventricles

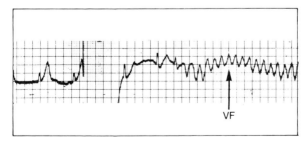

Figure 3.6   A ventricular ectopic falling on the T wave of the last sinus beat precipitates an attack of ventricular fibrillation

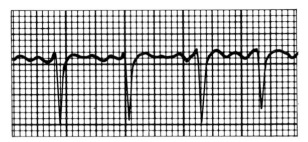

Figure 3.7   Atrial fibrillation

adults have frequent ventricular ectopic beats and, provided certain conditions are fulfilled, they can be safely ignored.

(1) There must be no clinical evidence of heart disease. The usual organic heart disease underlying ventricular ectopic beats is hypertension or myocardial ischemia.

(2) The electrocardiogram must be otherwise normal.

(3) Ectopic beats which are precipitated by exercise may be of some significance.

The following points should be looked for in the electro-cardiogram.

(a) Multifocal ectopics (i.e. ectopic beats with different patterns, Figure 3.5) and ectopics which occur in pairs are signs of organic heart disease.

(b) The T wave of the sinus beat following a benign ventricular ectopic should be identical to the preceding sinus beat. A change in the T wave following an ectopic beat suggests myocardial disease.

(c) Ectopic beats which are superimposed on the preceding sinus T wave should be regarded as pathological (Figure 3.6). Treatment is indicated only if there is underlying organic heart disease or if the patient is distressed by frequent palpitations. A number of effective drugs are available, for example, procainamide, quinidine, mex-iletine, disopyramide and the β blockers.

Atrial fibrillation. The typical irregularly irregular pulse of atrial fibrillation is an occasional unexpected finding and the diagnosis is readily confirmed by electrocardiography (Figure 3.7). Establishing the underlying etiology may be more difficult. Mitral valve disease, ischemic heart disease and hypertension account for the majority of cases and thyrotoxicosis for a few. Occasionally, no cause is found and the condition is then called 'lone atrial fibrillation'. Unexplained atrial fibrillation merits specialist advice, first, to clarify the etiology and second, because the use of anticoagulants or restoration of sinus rhythm by cardioversion may be indicated.

Bradycardia

Any patient with a heart rate of less than 60 beats per minute may be said to have a bradycardia, but a slow heart rate is not necessarily abnormal. Sinus bradycardia is common because it is a normal physiological response to increased vagal tone and, as such, is a feature of the simple faint (vasovagal syncope) and occurs in athletes. In addition, it is commonly induced by the β blocking drugs. It may, however, also be caused by degenerative changes in the sinoatrial node – a phenomenon which increases with age. Paradoxically, in some patients, sinus bradycardia alternates with paroxysms of tachycardia. This is a manifestation of the 'sick sinus syndrome'.

While minor degrees of bradycardia can be safely ignored, excessive slowing of the pulse (below 40 beats per minute) usually indicates that some degree of heart block is present. If no simple explanation for a symptomless bradycardia is apparent, an ECG will help to differentiate atrioventricular block from sinus bradycardia.

Heart block has many causes but in the context of the asymptomatic patient the etiology is almost invariably fibrosis and the conducting system. This appears to be a function of age and the majority of patients suffering from this condition are aged over 70 years. The association between a slow heart block, and dizziness or frank syncope (Stokes–Adams attacks) is well known. However, some patients have no symptoms at the time of diagnosis and remain asymptomatic for many years or indefinitely.

A permanent cardiac pacemaker is necessary for all patients with heart block who have any symptoms of dizziness or cardiac failure and is desirable for the elderly patient even if he is symptomless.

Blood pressure

Hypertension rarely causes symptoms until a catastrophe occurs, such as a cerebrovascular accident, cardiac failure or a myocardial infarction. Since it has been estimated that approximately 20% of the UK adult population has a blood pressure of 140/90 mmHg or more, and 5% of 150/105 mmHg or more, hypertension is found frequently on routine examination.

(1) If untreated, approximately 50% of patients with moderate hypertension die within five years. With adequate control the five year mortality is reduced to 15%.

(2) Adequate control of the blood pressure in patients with a diastolic pressure of 105 mmHg or more reduces the incidence of strokes by 75%, and markedly lessens the risk of cardiac failure and angina.

(3) All patients with hypertension should be screened, first, to assess the damage it has done, and second, to establish the etiology.

(4) Screening should include examination of urine for organisms, protein and glucose, blood urea and electrolyte estimation, electrocardiography and in some cases a chest X-ray and analysis of serum lipids.

(5) Treatment is indicated for patients with a diastolic pressure of 105 mmHg or more.

Auscultation of the heart

Practitioners in any branch of clinical medicine have to evaluate the significance of heart murmurs occasionally.

(1) Innocent murmurs, i.e. unassociated with disease or structural abnormality.

(2) Murmurs indicative of heart disease, which may or may not be serious.

(3) Physiological murmurs, such as those which occur during pregnancy or with anemia.

Heart murmurs in children

The size and nature of the problem created by unexpected murmurs is exemplified by the situation in children. It has been estimated that murmurs of no consequence can be heard in one third of all children. On the other hand, several significant congenital cardiac lesions are most often discovered at routine medical examinations, including aortic stenosis, pulmonary stenosis, atrial and ventricular septal defects and patent ductus arteriosus. Clearly, the need to differentiate between innocent and pathological murmurs is a common occurrence.

The following points permit the differentiation of innocent murmurs from those of a more serious nature.

(1) Innocent murmurs are always systolic, never diastolic.
(2) Innocent murmurs are of short duration and of no more than medium intensity.
(3) Innocent murmurs are unaccompanied by any other auscultatory abnormality.
(4) The patient with an innocent murmur is asymptomatic and has a normal electrocardiogram and chest X-ray.
(5) No other evidence of heart disease is present if the murmur is innocent.

The majority of innocent systolic murmurs in children fit into one of two groups.

Vibratory systolic murmur. Three quarters of all innocent murmurs are of this type. It is especially common in younger children and disappears at puberty. Maximal intensity is in the third and fourth left intercostal spaces. The murmur has been variously described as 'groaning', 'croaking', 'grating' and 'twanging'.

Pulmonic systolic murmur. This murmur is more common in adolescents and young adults. As the name suggests, it is maximal in the pulmonary area, but may radiate to the left sternal edge or apex. The murmur is short and blowing in character. A number of patients with this murmur will have either sternal depression or an abnormally straight back ('straight back syndrome').

A 'venous hum' is a continuous murmur superficially resembling the murmur of a patent ductus arteriosus. It is usually maximal above the clavicles. The pathognomonic feature which permits easy differentiation from patent ductus arteriosus is the fact that when the jugular vein is compressed above the auscultating stethoscope the murmur disappears, and also that the murmur changes markedly with differing positioning of the patient, being abolished in the head down position.

Specialist advice should be sought if the listed criteria are not fulfilled.

Heart murmurs in adults

Murmurs in adults are less often truly innocent but the same basic principles should be applied to establish their importance. That is, that the significance attached to a murmur depends to some extent on the associated findings, and the diastolic murmurs are usually pathological.

It should be remembered that, as in children, any condition associated with an increased cardiac output (anemia, thyrotoxicosis, fever and, specifically in adults, pregnancy) may produce a murmur while the condition persists.

Most murmurs discovered unexpectedly in adults are of one of two types.

Aortic ejection systolic murmur. We immediately think of aortic stenosis in this context, but in the middle-aged and elderly there are two much more common causes.

(1) Aortic sclerosis, i.e. thickening and fibrosis of the aortic valve.
(2) Dilatation of the ascending aorta associated with hypertension or arteriosclerosis.

These two conditions often occur together. It is not always easy to distinguish between these two causes and aortic stenosis, although careful attention to detail will provide the answer in most cases. Two important factors are first, that the character of the arterial pulse is usually altered in significant aortic stenosis – it is of low volume and slow rising, and second, that significant aortic stenosis is rare without some electrocardiographic evidence of left ventricular hypertrophy, although, of course, this may also be caused by hypertension. The safest course of action is to seek specialist advice if there is any doubt about the etiology of the murmur.

Mitral systolic murmur. In an asymptomatic adult, a mitral systolic murmur is usually due to one of two causes.

(1) A murmur confined to the latter part of systole is quite a common finding, especially in young women. It is often due to trivial mitral regurgitation caused by prolapse of a mitral valve cusp into the left atrium at the end of systole. Some authorities recommend that these patients should have anti-biotic prophylaxis for dental and other surgical procedures to reduce the risk of infective endocarditis.
(2) Fibrosis or calcification of the mitral valve ring is common in the elderly and produces the typical pansystolic murmur of mitral regurgitation.

ABNORMAL FINDINGS IN ROUTINE LABORATORY INVESTIGATIONS

Chest X-ray

Perhaps the most common unexpected finding is cardiomegaly. It is important to bear in mind that for an increased heart size to be apparent on X-ray considerable enlargement is necessary and that small increments on the radiograph reflect large changes in cardiac volume. Consequently, radiological evidence of an enlarged heart should always be taken seriously. The one exception to this rule is that in athletes, modest cardiomegaly is common. In adults, the cause is usually coronary artery disease or hypertension, but valvular disease and myocarditis are occasionally discovered in this way. If hypertension is the cause, routine investigations and treatment are indicated. In other situations, specialist advice should be sought.

Radiological abnormalities of the aorta caused by arterio-sclerosis increase with age. The changes produced in this way

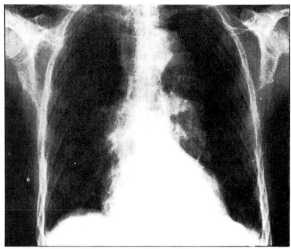

Figure 3.8   Chest radiograph of an 83-year-old man showing cardiac enlargement and aortic dilatation and unfolding

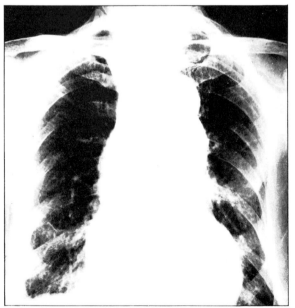

Figure 3.9   Calcification of aortic knuckle and of ascending aorta. There is aneurysmal dilatation of the descending thoracic aorta. This 75-year-old patient had no cardiac symptoms

include dilatation, unfolding (Figure 3.8) or tortuosity of the aorta and calcification of the aortic knuckle (Figure 3.9). In the elderly, such findings call for no specific action, but in younger patients the implied premature degenerative arterial disease can often be attributed to one of the known risk factors – notably hypertension, cigarette smoking and hyperlipidemia.

An abnormal chest radiograph will often confirm the presence of congenital heart disease in a child with an unexplained murmur. Even quite small intracardiac shunts (atrial or ventricular septal defects and patent ductus arteriosus) will cause pulmonary plethora, with or without cardiomegaly (Figure 3.10), and mild pulmonary stenosis causes bulging of the main pulmonary artery analogous to dilatation of the ascending aorta in aortic stenosis. It is worth remembering that since young children are unable to hold

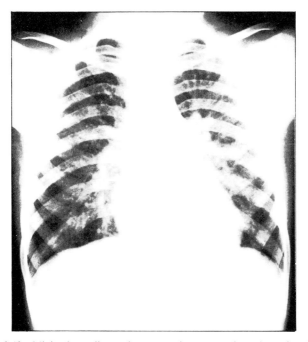

Figure 3.10 Minimal cardiac enlargement is present but there is obvious pulmonary plethora in this eight-year-old girl. A murmur was detected at routine medical examination. Cardiac catheterization confirmed the presence of a small atrial septal defect.

their breath in inspiration, the film may be taken during expiration which makes the heart appear larger.

Electrocardiogram

Abnormalities of rhythm. The most frequently encountered arrhythmias were discussed in the clinical section. The electrocardiogram is used to confirm the clinical diagnosis and for future reference.

Bundle branch block. Right bundle branch block is not rare. If the patient is a child, an atrial septal defect might be suspected, whereas in adults, hypertension and coronary artery disease are the commonest causes. In the elderly it often indicates fibrosis of the

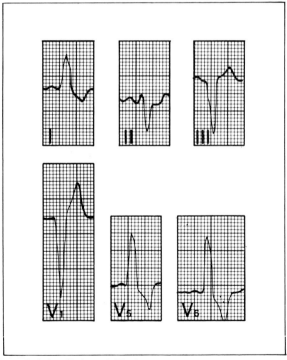

Figure 3.11   Left bundle branch block

conducting pathways and may progress to produce heart block. Left bundle branch block (Figure 3.11) is always regarded as pathological. It is usually caused by coronary artery disease.

Left ventricular hypertrophy. This is not an uncommon finding in asymptomatic patients with hypertension and indicates that the disease is seriously affecting the heart. If hypertension is not the cause, specialist advice should be sought as it probably indicates severe aortic valve disease or a cardiomyopathy.

Evidence of old myocardial infarction. The typical findings are of pathological Q waves with or without associated T wave inversion. 'Silent myocardial infarction' is a well-documented entity. If found, the patient should be assessed and investigated for the presence of risk factors which may be corrected.

Serum lipids

A wide variety of classifications has been proposed for the different abnormal lipid patterns which are encountered and this has led to a great deal of confusion. The need for different classifications has been brought about by the varied methods used to estimate the lipids in the blood. Simply stated however, each classification is designed to distinguish between abnormal elevations of cholesterol and triglycerides which occur alone or in combination. The best known classification is that devised by Fredrickson (Table 3.1), which describes five types of abnormality. Using his system, pure hypercholesterolemia is Type II and the commonly encountered combined elevation of cholesterol and triglyceride is Type IV.

The relationship between plasma lipids and atheroma is a complex one but from a practical point of view the essential facts are first, that ischemic heart disease occurs in more than half of all patients with Type II hyperlipidemia by the age of 50 years. Second, hypercholesterolemia increases the risk of developing ischemic heart disease by a factor of four. It would seem logical to deduce from this that reduction of plasma lipids would decrease the chances of developing ischemic heart disease. This has not been

Table 3.1 Classification of plasma lipid abnormalities (Fredrickson classification)

Fredrickson type	Lipid in excess	Comment and associations
I	Triglycerides	Very rare. Diagnosed in childhood
IIA	Cholesterol	Common. Increased incidence of coronary artery disease
IIB	Cholesterol and triglycerides	Common. Increased incidence of coronary diseases and diabetes
III	Cholesterol and triglycerides	Rare. Most have diabetes. Coronary and peripheral vascular disease common
IV and V	Triglycerides	Common (type IV). Obesity and diabetes common. Hyperuremia occurs. Coronary disease and hypertension are common

proved, but most authorities advise treatment to correct any lipid abnormality detected.

Treatment of hyperlipidemia

(1) Dietary restrictions may be imposed. A low animal fat diet can reduce the plasma cholesterol by 15 to 20%. Restriction of carbohydrate intake is effective in many patients with elevated triglycerides. Some authorities recommend that alcohol should be forbidden to patients with Type IV hyperlipidemia.

(2) The following drugs may be useful.

Cholestyramine. This ion exchange resin in a dose of 12 to 24 g per day can reduce plasma cholesterol by approximately 30%. Some patients find it unpalatable and constipation is quite common.

Clofibrate. 1.5 to 2.0 g per day can lower cholesterol by 10% and triglycerides by 20%.

Nicotinic acid is sometimes effective in lowering both cholesterol and triglyceride but side-effects, e.g. flushing, diarrhea and palpitations, are common.

Urea and electrolytes

In the absence of any other abnormal findings, deranged urea and electrolyte levels are unlikely to point to cardiovascular disease. When hypertension is present, however, a raised urea and/or potassium level may indicate renal disease as its cause. Rarely, electrolyte abnormalities may suggest Conn's syndrome or Cushing's syndrome.

Acknowledgement

Figures 3, 4, 5, 7, 11 and 12 taken from Fleming, J. S., *Interpreting the Electrocardiogram,* Update Books, London, 1979.

4

The Patient with Chest Pain

J. FLEMING and C. WARD

Is it angina? This thought often occurs to a patient when he first experiences pain in the chest and certainly occupies the mind of his general practitioner. Nothing can replace a careful history of the pain for diagnostic accuracy, and most mistakes in diagnosis occur as a result of proceeding too soon to the more impressive stages of examination and special investigations. The patient with angina usually appears completely normal on routine clinical examination and the resting electrocardiogram is normal. This is emphasized because many such patients are referred for an outpatient electro-cardiogram, and the unwary doctor may mistakenly reassure the patient on the basis of a normal report.

HISTORY TAKING AND EXAMINATION

The classical history of angina is a crushing retrosternal pain, per-haps spreading down the arms and up to the lower jaw (Figure 4.1), which comes on with exertion and obliges the patient to stop. The pain then subsides over the course of the next few minutes. Breath-lessness accompanies the pain but is not the dominant symptom. The amount of exertion undertaken before the occurrence of pain is not always constant and it is not unusual for a man to experience pain walking to work in the morning and thereafter to perform quite heavy physical work without further discomfort. It is the relationship of chest pain to exertion which is the most crucial feature in reaching the diagnosis of angina pectoris. The precise

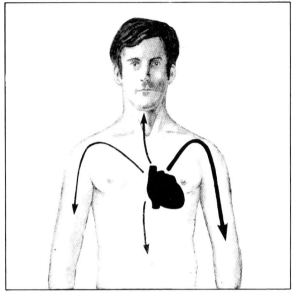

Figure 4.1   Typical distribution of pain in angina pectoris

nature of the pain is not so important: patients describe it variously as vice-like, burning, heavy or like toothache and some patients are unable to give an adequate description at all. If, however, the words 'sharp', 'like a knife' or 'stabbing' are used then there is a distinct possibility that the diagnosis is not angina. The young man who describes a sharp stab of momentary duration in the region of the left breast, which bears no relation to exertion, is not suffering from angina.

When the history is typical then the diagnosis of angina pectoris is made at this stage before proceeding to clinical examination. By far the commonest cause for angina is, of course, atheroma affecting the coronary arteries. No evidence of this is to be found on clinical examination. Nevertheless a clinical examination is essential to rule out other less common causes of angina, such as severe aortic valve disease, and to detect any conditions which aggravate angina, e.g. anemia, obesity and hypertension.

INVESTIGATIONS

In the typical case of angina investigations are undertaken as an aid to management rather than as a means of diagnosis. A resting electrocardiogram is not essential but may be useful for comparison with any electrocardiograms recorded in the future should complications develop such as myocardial infarction. An exercise electrocardiogram will not add to the diagnosis nor aid in management and should not be requested. Estimation of the fasting serum cholesterol and triglycerides will detect any gross lipid abnormality and should be undertaken in young and middle-aged patients with angina. Values tend to fluctuate in the individual patient, partly because there may be quite large variations caused by seasonal changes, drugs, change of diet and changes in body weight and partly because of laboratory factors. Fasting serum lipid studies should be obtained on two or three separate occasions before

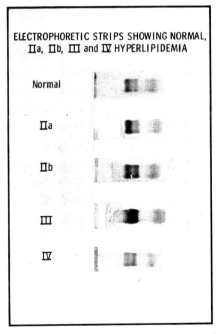

Figure 4.2 Normal and abnormal electrophoretic patterns in hyperlipidemia (Fredrickson's classification)

attempting to diagnose a disorder of lipid metabolism. An abnormality of serum lipids will be detected in 30% of patients with angina and will lead to appropriate dietary drug measures for its correction (Figure 4.2).

Familial hypercholesterolemia is common, comprising 45 to 55% of all abnormal lipoprotein patterns. Typically, there is a family history of coronary artery disease, a corneal arcus is seen and a xanthoma may be detectable on palpation of the Achilles tendon. Serum cholesterol is greatly increased and the triglycerides are normal.

Carbohydrate-induced hyperlipidemia is also common. In addition to obesity these patients frequently have diabetes mellitus and hyperuricemia. The serum cholesterol is high, the serum triglycerides are moderately increased and the glucose tolerance test is abnormal.

The important protective effect of the high density lipoproteins is now recognized. A high level of these lipoproteins aids in the tissue mobilization of cholesterol, and the presence of a high serum cholesterol is probably much less dangerous if there is an accompanying high concentration of high density lipoproteins. Estimation of these lipoproteins should be undertaken in addition to serum cholesterol and triglycerides. Any suspicion of anemia or thyroid disorder would require a full blood count and estimation of serum thyroxine, serum T3 uptake and perhaps serum TSH.

MANAGEMENT

General

The majority of patients with angina pectoris are managed exclusively by the general practitioner and lead active lives (Figure 4.3). A weight reducing diet is often necessary and cigarette smoking should be forbidden. Most patients will continue with their work but those doing a strenuous job will find their capacity limited by the onset of pain and may have to seek lighter work. Drivers of public service and heavy goods vehicles and airline pilots must inform the appropriate authorities and take up more suitable work where any sudden illness would not be a hazard to the general

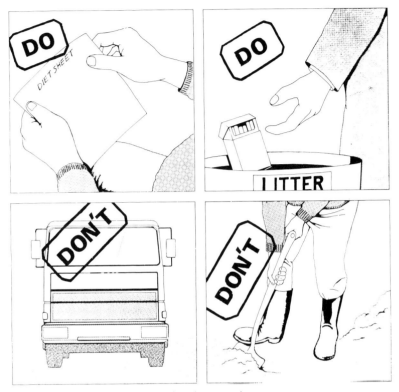

Figure 4.3 General management of angina pectoris

public. There is no prohibition from driving private vehicles except when angina is easily provoked during driving.

Physical exercise up to, but not beyond, the onset of chest pain is encouraged and may stimulate the growth of a collateral coronary circulation. The patient is provided with glyceryl trinitrate 0.5 mg tablets and encouraged to chew one not only at the onset of pain but also whenever undertaking exertion likely to provoke pain. Sudden bursts of strenuous exertion may be dangerous, for example, shovelling snow from the driveway in winter, running to catch a train while carrying a heavy suitcase, or playing squash. Golf provides a more gentle sport and tennis need not be forbidden.

Beta-blockade

The beta-blocking drugs reduce the work load on the heart by slowing the heart rate and lowering the blood pressure. The exercise tolerance of most patients with angina is significantly improved by the use of these drugs and the general practitioner should prescribe the beta-blocker he is most familiar with as there is little to choose between the wide variety available for the management of angina. A small initial dose is advised because undesirable side-effects, such as bronchospasm, may appear. The beta-blocking drugs are probably best avoided for the patient with a history of asthma, but if pain is difficult to control then a cardioselective drug should be preferred. There is a possibility that a beta-blocking drug will intensify any heart failure or any tendency to bradycardia, so hospital outpatient referral is recommended for the patient with bradycardia, a large heart or evidence of heart failure. In some of these patients a beta-blocking drug may be beneficial after giving digoxin.

The maximum benefit in angina is obtained with moderately large dosage of the beta-blocker so that an initial dosage of 40 mg t.d.s. of propranolol can be increased to 80 mg t.d.s., then to 160 mg b.d. if symptoms are not adequately controlled. Side-effects which, if mild, need not lead to discontinuation of the drug, include a feeling of tiredness, cold extremities and vivid dreams at night. Abrupt cessation of therapy should be avoided as there is evidence that myocardial infarction may be precipitated. The presence of diabetes mellitus is not an absolute contraindication to the use of beta-blocking drugs but particular care is required for the patient receiving insulin because the beta-blocking drugs interfere with the defence reactions against hypoglycemia. A more selective beta-blocker should be prescribed for such patients.

Blood lipid abnormalities

No dramatic benefit will result from the discovery and treatment of abnormalities of the blood fats in the patient with angina because to a large extent the damage has already been done. However, perhaps further accumulation of cholesterol in the intima of the coronary arteries may be prevented. There is no clear evidence that a reduction in size of cholesterol plaques in the coronary arteries is brought about by cholesterol-lowering regimes, and clinical trials have not yet provided convincing proof of any effect on prognosis. Nevertheless, most clinicians agree that treatment is desirable for any identified lipid disorder, the vigour with which the treatment is pursued depending on the patient's individual circumstances. A young patient with a very high cholesterol level potentially stands to gain much more from treatment than a 70-year-old patient in the same condition. Abnormalities of lipid metabolism may be secondary to identifiable disease such as diabetes mellitus, hypo-thyroidism, nephrotic syndrome, biliary obstruction and pan-creatitis. It is more common that the hyperlipidemia is a 'primary' abnormality (due to genetically determined defects in lipid metabolism which are exaggerated by environmental factors) in which case therapy is directed towards appropriate modification of the diet, supplemented in some patients by drug therapy.

The diet for patients with familial hypercholesterolemia should provide less than 300 mg of cholesterol per day and contain twice as much polyunsaturated fat as saturated fat. If, after a few months of this diet, the fall in serum cholesterol is less than 10% then nicotinic acid or clofibrate may be added. Nicotinic acid is required in a dosage of 1 g three times daily after meals, but commencing at smaller dosage levels to minimize cutaneous flushing. Other side-effects of nicotinic acid are abdominal discomfort and an increased level of uric acid and blood sugar. Clofibrate is given in a dosage of 1 g twice daily and has few side-effects apart from a tendency to cause diarrhea. For the patients with carbohydrate induced hyperlipidemia a weight reducing diet containing equal proportions of polyunsaturated and saturated fats is prescribed. Refined sugar should be avoided and the daily cholesterol intake restricted to 300 to 500 mg.

PROGNOSIS

The prognosis is good for the patient with stable angina and many learn to live with their limitations and lead a normal life. Life expectancy may not necessarily be severely decreased, particularly if the coronary artery disease is not extensive. Unfortunately, the number and sites of coronary arteries blocked in each patient can only be determined by coronary arteriography, and since this investigation is reserved for selected cases we cannot give a precise prognosis. A change in the pattern of the angina may give warning of an impending infarction.

Despite good medical treatment a number of patients remain severely limited in their exercise tolerance and in this group coronary arteriography (Figure 4.4) followed by coronary artery bypass surgery may prove successful. The usual indication for coronary arteriography is the patient with severe angina pectoris which is unresponsive to medical treatment and in whom coronary artery surgery is under consideration. The upper age limit is about 65 years and left ventricular function must be good. The patient is admitted to hospital for coronary arteriography, which carries a risk of one serious complication per 1,000 investigations per-

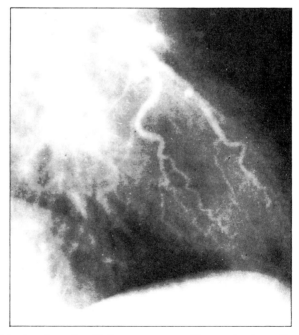

Figure 4.4   Arteriography of left coronary artery. The anterior descending artery is occluded

formed, and surgery will be offered if the left ventricular angiogram shows a good ventricle and the coronary arteries distal to the obstruction are not severely diseased. As many as four saphenous vein bypass grafts may be inserted during the operation (Figure 4.5). The risk of death during surgery is about 2 to 3% and after surgery over 80% of patients are improved, a substantial proportion being completely asymptomatic (Figure 4.6). Late deterioration due to subsequent thrombosis of the saphenous vein graft may occur in 15 to 20% of patients.

There is yet no universal agreement concerning the place of coronary artery surgery in the management of the patient with angina. Some patients do have incapacitating angina despite good medical therapy and the prospect of amelioration or complete relief from pain following successful surgery would indicate to many physicians that surgery should be considered in this group. At least they will be improved symptomatically. The strong advocates of coronary artery surgery also believe that the prognosis is favourably influenced, particularly when there is severe stenosis of the left main stem coronary artery. At present there is no clear evidence that life expectancy is improved by coronary artery surgery and many physicians do not believe that it can be expected to prolong life.

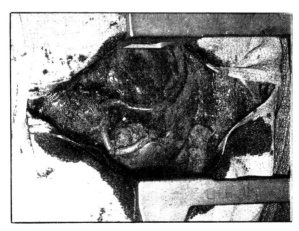

Figure 4.5   Operative photograph showing two saphenous vein grafts in position (courtesy of E. J. M. Weaver)

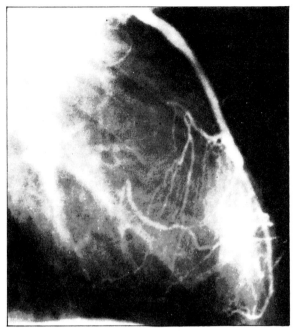

Figure 4.6 Postoperative angiogram showing successful vein graft. Contrast has been injected down the saphenous graft which fills the anterior descending artery

DIAGNOSTIC PROBLEMS

The majority of patients with coronary artery disease causing angina are sufficiently typical to be clearly diagnosed and managed by the general practitioner. Some patients with pain thought to be cardiac in origin present real difficulties in diagnosis when, for example, the pain is prolonged, poorly related to exertion and not relieved by sublingual glyceryl trinitrate. These patients will probably be referred to the hospital outpatient clinic where initial investigations will include electrocardiography at rest and with exercise. The electrocardiogram is recorded during and immediately after submaximal or maximal exertion under strictly controlled conditions in the cardiac laboratory (Figure 4.7). The results are not always easy to interpret because the characteristic abnormality seen in angina pectoris is a depression of the ST seg-

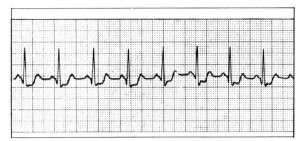

Figure 4.7 Electrocardiogram of positive exercise tests. The exercise was not strenuous, the heart rate reaching 100 beats per minute. The ST segment is depressed 2 mm, and the ST depression in this patient is of the typical horizontal shape of myocardial ischemia

ment and the ST segment deviation is difficult to see when the baseline of the electrocardiogram is not steady. Furthermore, if we use as our criterion a 2 mm ST segment depression, we will miss many cases of coronary artery disease. Acceptance of lesser degrees of ST segment deviation will lead to fewer cases being missed but may involve a considerable number of false positive diagnoses being made. Whatever criteria are chosen for the interpretation of the exercise electrocardiogram, about 30% of patients with coronary artery disease will show a normal result. The exercise electrocardiogram is a useful test when the patient has undiagnosed chest pain, but has severe limitations. A normal exercise electrocardiogram does not rule out coronary artery disease.

Coronary arteriography

There may be a place for coronary arteriography as an aid to diagnosis, particularly when, for example, the patient's livelihood is threatened. This investigation cannot always be regarded as diagnostic because some patients apparently have normal coronary arteries yet suffer from angina pectoris and may even subsequently die from myocardial infarction. The explanation is not known and suggestions range from the postulate that there is disease of the small coronary branches or of the myocardial cells, to the fairly well substantiated hypothesis that transient severe spasm may occur in a major coronary artery. There is the additional problem of interpretation of the coronary arteriogram when an obstructive lesion is seen. Not all obstructions are clinically significant and care must be exercised before making the assumption that an abnormality seen on the coronary angiogram is the cause of the patient's chest pain.

The Prinzmetal variant

The Prinzmetal variant of angina pectoris (Figure 4.8) is not common but may cause much difficulty in diagnosis. The underlying pathology appears to be transient spasm of a coronary artery in some cases and severe stenosis of a main coronary artery in others. Bouts of chest pain occur at rest and often last for several hours, with the electrocardiogram showing ST segment elevation during the attack, as opposed to the usual appearance during angina of ST depression. Suspected cases are investigated in hospital with continuous electrocardiographic recordings and, during coronary arteriography, if the coronary arteries appear normal,

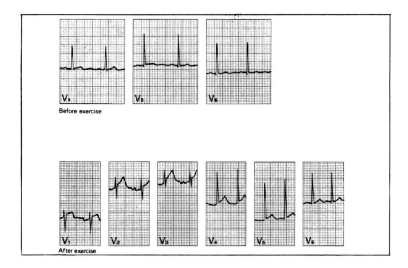

Figure 4.8 Exercise test showing Prinzmetal's angina. Before the exercise V_4, V_5 and V_6 are seen to be within normal limits. After exercise there is ST segment elevation in precordial leads V_1 to V_5

attempts may be made to induce spasm in a coronary artery by the injection of drugs.

Other causes of chest pain

Finally, there are, of course, many other causes of chest pain unrelated to the coronary vessels or to the heart. Pleuritic pain is

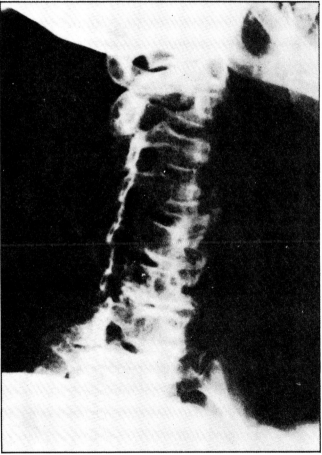

Figure 4.9 Cervical spondylosis. Oblique radiograph showing oesteophytic encroachment on intervertebral foramina at C5/C6 and C6/C7 levels

usually easily identified by the sharpness of the pain and by the relation to respiration. Acid reflux causing esophagitis may be more difficult to diagnose and the pain of cervical spondylosis (Figure 4.9) can mimic many of the features of angina. In most cases the key features – the relationship of the pain to exercise and emotion, the site and radiation of the pain and the effect of glyceryl trinitrate – will enable the differentiation to be made between angina and chest pain of other cause.

Acknowledgement

We would like to thank Dr Alistair McDonald for permission to reproduce Figures 4.4, 4.5 and 4.6.

5
Hypertension

C. WARD and J. FLEMING

There is no clear-cut dividing line between what is a normal and what is an abnormal blood pressure. A blood pressure which is apparently harmless to one person may be harmful to another. Nevertheless, to facilitate discussion and treatment it is necessary to set an upper limit of normality. The consensus of opinion is that a blood pressure greater than 140/90 mmHg should be regarded as abnormal – but not necessarily as an indication for treatment. Blood pressure tends to rise with increasing age and women appear to tolerate an elevated blood pressure better than men. It remains to be seen whether or not it is justifiable to infer from this that a higher blood pressure is normal in the elderly or in women than in young men.

INCIDENCE OF HYPERTENSION

Estimates of the incidence of hypertension will depend on criteria for diagnosis, the technique of measurement, the circumstances under which it is recorded and the population being studied. However, the following approximate figures indicate the size of the problem in the UK: 5% of the adult population have a diastolic pressure greater than 110 mmHg, and 15 to 20% have a diastolic pressure of 90 to 110 mmHg.

CAUSES OF HYPERTENSION

We have learned a lot recently about the normal regulation of the blood pressure, but the underlying mechanism of hypertension is still not known. The blood pressure reflects the tone in the peripheral arterioles and the elasticity of the large arteries. The kidneys play a major role in its control through the renin-angiotensin system (Figure 5.1). The most plausible theory so far is that hyper-

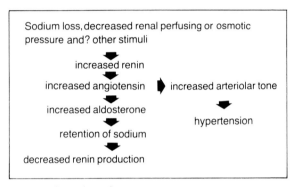

Figure 5.1   The renin-angiotensin system

tension is caused by increased sensitivity to normal amounts of angiotensin II (or other pressor amines such as adrenaline). The increased arteriolar tone which this causes is reversible at first but later becomes fixed. This eventually results in hypertrophy of the muscle layers of larger arteries which subsequently undergo degenerative changes. When elevation of the blood pressure is marked, the process becomes self-perpetuating and may cause the changes of malignant hypertension. The hallmark of this condition is fibrinoid necrosis in which damage to the endothelial lining of arterioles leads to extravasation of fibrin and blood into the media causing tissue damage.

IMPORTANCE OF HYPERTENSION

Whatever the underlying mechanism, the essential facts are that hypertension produces degenerative arterial changes and that these

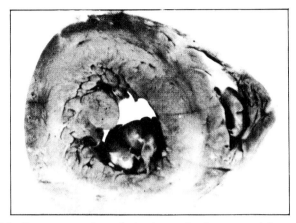

Figure 5.2 Transverse section of the heart showing severe left ventricular hypertrophy caused by long-standing hypertension

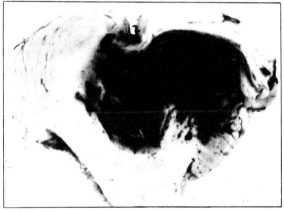

Figure 5.3 Massive intracerebral hemorrhage in a middle-aged patient with hypertension who had been asymptomatic until he collapsed 48 hours before death

changes seriously affect the function of vital organs – in particular the heart (Figure 5.2), the brain (Figure 5.3) and the kidneys (Figure 5.4). It is important to appreciate that hypertension is only one of several factors which are known to cause degenerative arterial disease: hyperlipidemia, diabetes mellitus, cigarette smoking and genetic factors also play a part. There is also evidence

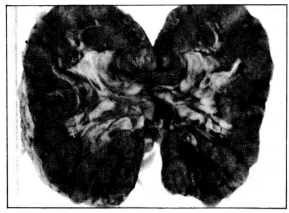

Figure 5.4 The kidney in long-standing hypertension. The cortex is narrowed and the outline is markedly irregular

of an increased prevalence of hyperuricemia in both renal and essential hypertension. The deleterious effects of a particular blood pressure are accentuated by the presence of any of these factors.

Hypertension reduces life expectancy as a result of coronary artery disease, strokes, renal failure, cardiac failure and peripheral vascular disease. These complications do not suddenly occur at a specific level of blood pressure. Their incidence increases in proportion to the degree of hypertension and to the presence of risk factors.

Data from major life insurance companies (Figure 5.5) clearly show that relatively minor elevations of blood pressure are harmful and that prognosis worsens progessively as blood pressure rises (Metropolitan Life Insurance Co. 1961). It is not only the diastolic blood pressure which is important. At any given diastolic pressure the mortality rises in proportion to the systolic pressure.

Two specific statistics serve to show that hypertension is a major health hazard: a) the life expectancy of a young man with a blood pressure of 150/110mmHg is reduced by more than 15 years, and b) untreated, the five-year mortality of moderate hypertension is approximately 50%.

The importance of detecting hypertension at an early stage lies in the knowledge that treatment dramatically reduces complications and thus improves the prognosis.

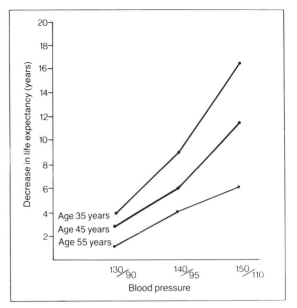

Figure 5.5 The effect of blood pressure on life expectancy at different ages

AETIOLOGY

In 95% of cases no cause for the hypertension can be found. This is essential hypertension. The remaining 5% of cases are grouped together as secondary hypertension. One of the aims of investigating the hypertensive patient is to establish whether the hypertension is essential or secondary, because in some cases secondary hypertension can be cured by appropriate surgery – an attractive alternative to life-long drug therapy.

Secondary hypertension

Renal disease

Almost any type of renal disease can cause hypertension. Pyelonephritis, hydronephrosis and renal stones rarely cause severe hypertension probably because they do not stimulate renin secretion. Not only does renal disease cause hypertension but, of course, hypertension causes renal damage. When the hypertension is secondary to renal disease the elevated blood pressure may initiate a vicious cycle by causing further deterioration in the already poor renal function. The importance of detecting a renal cause for hypertension is threefold.

(1) If the renal disease is unilateral (e.g. see Figure 5.6), removal of the affected kidney may affect a cure.
(2) The over-enthusiastic treatment of hypertension in the presence of pre-existing renal disease may cause further deterioration in renal function.
(3) Occasionally, in advanced renal failure, the blood pressure can only be controlled after nephrectomy.

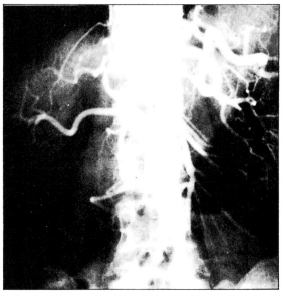

Figure 5.6 Aortography showing the radiological changes of renal artery stenosis

Endocrine Causes

There are three major endocrine disorders which cause hypertension. Each is due to an abnormality of the adrenal glands – either hyperplasia or a tumour.

Cushing's syndrome. The underlying abnormality in Cushing's syndrome is usually increased secretion of ACTH by the pituitary gland which in turn stimulates excess production of cortisol by the adrenal cortices. Occasionally the cause is an adrenal tumour. Hypertension occurs in more than 75% of cases.

Phaeochromocytoma. This is a rare tumour of the adrenal medulla which secretes excess adrenaline and noradrenaline causing paroxysmal hypertension with paroxysms of headache and palpitations. Glycosuria and weight loss are usually present.

Primary hyperaldosteronism (Conn's syndrome). In this condition an adrenal adenoma produces an excess of the hormone aldosterone, causing mild hypertension.

Coarctation of the Aorta

Coarctation of the aorta is a congenital narrowing of the upper part of the descending aorta which causes hypertension and rib notching, which is visible on the chest radiograph. It carries a poor prognosis if untreated.

Drugs

ACTH and steroids. The therapeutic administration of these agents has the same effect on the blood pressure as does Cushing's syndrome. The blood pressure of patients receiving these drugs should be checked regularly.

The contraceptive pill. Oral contraceptives occasionally cause hypertension. The blood pressure should be recorded before 'the pill' is prescribed, and checked from time to time thereafter. If an elevation in blood pressure is noted, cessation of the drug usually results in the return of the blood pressure to normal over the course of a few weeks or months. Oral contraceptives should not be prescribed for known hypertensive patients.

Others. Hypertension is occasionally caused by carbenoxolone or proprietary cold cures which contain sympathomimetic amines.

DIAGNOSIS AND ASSESSMENT

The two most important facts relating to hypertension are first, that it rarely causes symptoms until a catastrophe occurs and second, that treatment dramatically improves the prognosis (Figure 5.7). The implications are clear: hypertension should be diagnosed and treated before complications occur.

Patients with a diastolic blood pressure of 90 to 100 mmHg should have it checked several times over the course of a few months. If the initial reading is confirmed, the patient should be reviewed regularly, perhaps once or twice a year. As a general guideline, all patients with an established diastolic pressure of more than 100 mmHg should be carefully assessed, although not necessarily treated. It is to these patients that the following suggestions on management particularly apply.

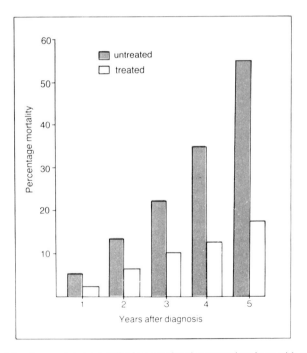

Figure 5.7 Accumulated mortality in treated and untreated patients with moderate hypertension

The examination of patients with hypertension has three objectives: to assess its severity, to detect the presence of other factors which cause arterial disease and thus accentuate the effects of hypertension, and to determine whether the hypertension is essential or secondary.

The History

Although hypertension remains symptomless for many years, patients should be carefully questioned on specific points. Breathlessness, angina or visual disturbances indicate, if caused by hypertension, that it is well advanced. In particular, visual disturbances may be due to malignant hypertension which requires urgent hospitalization. Patients should also be asked about current drug therapy and smoking habits.

Patients with essential hypertension usually know of family members with coronary artery disease, strokes, peripheral vascular disease or elevated blood pressure. The absence of such a family history suggests that their hypertension may be secondary.

The patient should be asked if his blood pressure has been taken in the past and if any comment was made. Practice records, hospital correspondence and insurance or medical reports are checked: a recent significant blood pressure change often denotes secondary hypertension.

Intermittent attacks of pallor, flushing, palpitations, headaches and anxiety suggest phaeochromocytoma.

Examination

General features. The triad of obesity, abdominal striae and hirsutism is found in Cushing's syndrome and in steroid therapy. Neurofibromatosis is a rare indication of phaeochromocytoma.

Auscultation and palpation. An aortic systolic murmur may be heard when the valve is sclerosed or in coarctation of the aorta. A gallop rhythm is an indication of impending cardiac failure. Displacement of the apex beat to the left is an indication of left ventricular enlargement.

Peripheral pulses. The leg pulses should be assessed for evidence of peripheral vascular disease. More specifically, absence or delay of the femoral pulses is almost pathognomonic of coarctation of the aorta.

Abdominal examination. It is important to try to assess the size of the kidneys. If both are enlarged it suggests either polycystic kidneys (Figure 5.8) or bilateral hydronephrosis. If one kidney is larger than the other, unilateral renal disease is present. The detection of an abdominal bruit by auscultating just above the umbilicus suggests renal artery stenosis.

The optic fundi. Ophthalmoscopy should be an integral part of the examination of all patients with hypertension: it permits direct visualization of small arteries and gives an indication of the damage which the patient's hypertension has caused. The changes have been graded and reflect the severity of the hypertension.

Grade 1. Calibre of arterioles significantly less than that of their accompanying veins.

Grade 2. Irregularity of arteriolar lumen.

Grade 3. Hemorrhages and exudates. The hemorrhages are either

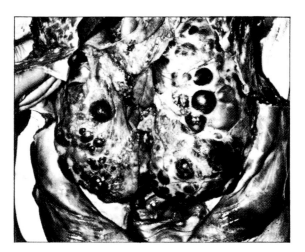

Figure 5.8 Polycystic kidneys at postmortem

flame-shaped or like blots. The exudates are described as 'cotton wool' because of their fuzzy outline.

Grade 4. Papilledema. Its presence indicates malignant hypertension – although malignant hypertension may be present without papilledema.

Investigations

The investigation of patients with hypertension should be undertaken with the same aims in mind as the examination, i.e. to assess severity, to discover other risk factors and to determine whether the hypertension is essential or secondary. All the necessary investigations can be performed at or from the practice surgery and should form part of the routine assessment of all hypertensive patients.

Urea, electrolytes and uric acid. An elevated blood urea indicates probable renal impairment and in essential hypertension it shows that the elevated blood pressure has seriously affected renal function. Hypokalemia and alkalosis may indicate Conn's syndrome but are more often caused by previous diuretic therapy. Raised uric acid may be associated with both renal and essential hypertension, and may also occur following diuretic therapy.

Hemoglobin Estimation

Urine. A urine sample should be sent with details to the laboratory for bacteriological culture. A further specimen should be tested for glucose and protein. In the absence of malignant hypertension, significant proteinuria indicates intrinsic renal disease.

Electrocardiogram. The electrocardiogram becomes progressively more abnormal as the heart becomes hypertrophied in response to hypertension (Figure 5.9).

Plasma lipids. Plasma lipids are estimated in younger patients. At any given level of blood pressure, the risks of developing arterial disease are increased by hyperlipidemia.

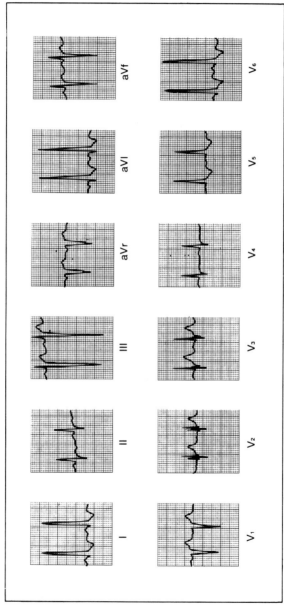

Figure 5.9 Electrocardiogram of a 56-year-old asymptomatic lady with a blood pressure of 240/140 mmHg and Grade III retinopathy. Marked left ventricular hypertrophy is indicated by increased QRS voltages in the anterolateral leads and by left ventricular strain pattern

Chest X-ray. Cardiomegaly is a precursor of cardiac failure and indicates serious cardiac involvement. The radiograph may also show the typical features of coarctation of the aorta.

TREATMENT

The aims of treatment are first, to reduce the blood pressure to normal or near normal levels so that the risk of complications is decreased or removed, and second, to prevent the recurrence or progression of complications which have already occurred.

In order to justify life-long drug therapy for hypertensive patients, many of whom will be asymptomatic, it is clearly necessary to show that treatment is beneficial. The evidence which forms a rational basis for deciding which patients should be treated can be summarized as follows:

(1) Before the advent of effective therapy the mortality for malignant hypertension at two years was 90%. Nowadays, once the malignant phase has been reversed, the prognosis is the same as for other patients with comparable blood pressure.

(2) The adequate control of blood pressure in patients with a diastolic pressure of more than 105 mmHg results in minimal risk of developing heart failure, the relief or marked reduction of angina in 50% of patients and a 75% reduction in the incidence of strokes.

(3) A large scale study in the USA has shown that in young and middle-aged men the control of moderate hypertension (diastolic pressure of more than 114 mmHg) reduces the five-year mortality from more than 50% to approximately 15% (The Veterans Administration Co-operative Study Group 1967).

Thus the case for treating *all* patients with a diastolic pressure of more than 105 mmHg is strong. Objective grounds for treating patients with lesser degrees of hypertension (i.e. a blood pressure of around 140/90 mmHg) may come from current studies. However, if a patient has evidence of arterial disease or if other risk factors are present, treatment may be justified.

Two further points should be noted, which are contrary to past teaching. First, the elderly stand to benefit from treatment: therapy should not be withheld purely on the basis of age. The aim in the elderly should be to reduce the blood pressure modestly and gradually, taking particular care to avoid postural hypotension.

Second, a previous stroke or a history of myocardial infarction should no longer be considered to contraindicate treatment. These patients gain as much from adequate therapy as any others.

The large number of preparations available for treating hypertension has given rise to a wide variety of recommended treatment schedules. Although there is no one correct regimen the objective should always be to achieve optimum reduction of blood pressure with a minimum of tablets and side-effects. The regimen outlined below is widely used and it is effective in about 90% of cases seen in general practice.

Suggested treatment schedule

Diastolic pressure 105 to 115 mmHg

Many patients can be adequately treated with a long-acting diuretic such as a thiazide or chlorthalidone, but the following precautions should be borne in mind:

(1) Hypokalemia may occur and the serum potassium should be checked after a few weeks of treatment. To avoid hypokalemia, several diuretic combinations have been introduced, one component of which has a potassium-retaining action. e.g. spironolactone with hydroflumethiazide, triamterene with hydrochlorothiazide and amiloride with hydrochlorothiazide.

(2) Diabetes may be caused or worsened. The thiazides are therefore best avoided in diabetes.

(3) Most diuretics can cause hyperuricemia and may precipitate an acute attack of gout. They should not be prescribed for patients known to have gout unless there is no suitable alternative.

Diastolic pressure of more than 115 mmHg (or failure of diuretic alone)

In this situation a beta-blocker in combination with a long-acting diuretic should be given. The beta-blockers are very effective hypotensive agents. They have one major advantage over other drugs of comparable potency in that they do not cause postural hypotension. The major contraindications to the use of beta-blockers are cardiac failure and obstructive airways disease. For most patients, all beta-blockers are equally effective, although specific circumstances may affect the choice as follows:

(1) Most beta-blockers potentiate the effects of insulin and of hypoglycemic agents. Metoprolol may be less likely to do this than others. All diabetics who are prescribed a beta-blocker should be carefully observed.

(2) Occasionally, patients will complain of sedation, vivid dreams, mood changes or even hallucinations. Beta-blockers which do not cross the blood-brain barrier (such as sotalol or metoprolol) are less likely to cause these complications.

(3) Some patients complain of cold feet. It has been suggested that propranolol is more likely to cause this than are other beta-blockers.

(4) Patient compliance may be more likely with a once-daily beta-blocker such as atenalol.

(5) The optimum dosage of propranolol varies more widely than that of other beta-blockers. Consequently, treatment may need adjustment during follow-up.

If, for any reason, a beta-blocker is contraindicated, methyldopa is a suitable alternative.

Failure of diuretic plus beta-blocker

If the blood pressure remains high despite adequate dosage of a beta-blocker with a long-acting diuretic, hydralazine should be added. This drug has gained notoriety because in high dosage it occasionally causes systemic lupus erythematosus: in the dose now recommended (25 to 50 mg t.i.d.) this is rare. A recently introduced alternative vasodilator is prazosin.

Other Drugs

Methyldopa. This remains one of the most widely used hypotensive agents. It is very effective and produces a gradual reduction of blood pressure. However, compared with the beta-blockers, side-effects are common, e.g. postural hypotension, fatigue and sedation.

Guanethidine, bethanidine and debrisoquine. These drugs are postganglionic sympathetic neurone blockers. They are potent hypotensive agents which may be tried if other treatment fails. Their major drawback is the high incidence of unpleasant side-effects, such as postural hypotension, failure of ejaculation and diarrhea.

Labetalol. This drug, which has a combination of alpha- and beta-blocking actions, has recently been introduced. It is a promising addition to the available drugs but is still undergoing long-term assessment.

Referral to Hospital

The majority of hypertensive patients can be investigated and treated by their family doctor. Occasionally, however, it will be necessary to refer patients to hospital either for investigation or urgent treatment.

Special investigations. When the history, examination or routine investigations suggest that the patient may have secondary hypertension, referral to a hospital outpatient clinic is indicated. For patients with suspected renal disease, an intravenous pyelogram may be all that is necessary. In other cases, renal arteriography, radio-active isotope scanning or other specialized investigations may be required. Patients with coarctation of the aorta should be hospitalized for angiography and surgery. When an endocrine disorder is suspected, hospitalization is usually required for metabolic studies and for serum and urinary hormone assays.

Treatment. Hospitalization is indicated either for urgent reduction of the blood pressure or for careful monitoring in three situations:

(1) Malignant hypertension. There is no specific level of blood pressure at which malignant hypertension can be said to occur. However, the diastolic pressure will almost invariably be greater than 120 mmHg and is usually much higher. It is usually accompanied by papilledema or hemorrhages and exudates. Rapid controlled reduction in blood pressure is needed to prevent irreversible arterial damage.

(2) Hypertensive encephalopathy. This is probably caused by cerebral edema. The main clinical features are headache and confusion which may progress to stupor, fits or coma. It should be noted that hypertensive encephalopathy is rare, and that the features noted are more often due to some other cause.

(3) Hypertensive heart failure. In this situation, treatment is required for both the heart failure and the hypertension.

Follow-up

A variety of programmes have been recommended for the follow-up of hypertensive patients. Whatever scheme is adopted, the aims should be to check the blood pressure of as many adult patients as possible every few years, to ensure that the blood pressure of patients on treatment is adequately controlled and to recheck patients with borderline blood pressures at regular intervals.

Hypertensive therapy is now so effective (although not ideal) that the occurrence of complications should be regarded as a failure of our screening or treatment and not as an inevitable consequence of the disease. The following guidelines will cover most eventualities:

(1) If blood pressure is normal, recheck after four or five years.

(2) Patients with a diastolic blood pressure of 90 to 110 mmHg should be checked in six to eight weeks.
      If the level has fallen, recheck every six to twelve months. If the diastolic pressure remains about 105 mmHg, commence treatment.

(3) Patients on treatment should be seen every three to four months.

References

The Veterans Administration Co-operative Study Group on Anti-hypertensive Agents, 1967, *J. Am. Med. Assoc.*, **202**, 1028.

Metropolitan Life Insurance Co., 1961, *Blood Pressure: Insurance Experience and its Implications,* New York

6
Cardiac Arrhythmias

C. WARD and J. FLEMING

With the exception of ectopic beats, the common arrhythmias can be divided into tachycardias (heart rate above 100 beats per minute) and bradycardias (heart rate below 60 beats per minute). The tachycardias are sub-divided into supraventricular and ventricular (Table 6.1).

Table 6.1   Classification of common arrhythmias

Tachycardias

a) Supraventricular
   Sinus tachycardia
   Paroxysmal atrial tachycardia
   Nodal tachycardia
   Atrial flutter
   Atrial fibrillation

b) Ventricular tachycardia

Bradycardias

a) Sinus bradycardia
b) Sino-atrial block
c) Atrioventricular block

THE HISTORY

A carefully taken history will often give a clue to the nature of arrhythmia (Table 6.2). At the same time the following points must be kept in mind:

(1) Arrhythmias produce a variety of symptoms, not all of

Table 6.2 Diagnosis of arrhythmias – clues from the history

Clue	Possible diagnosis
1. Onset in infancy/ childhood	Paroxysmal atrial tachycardia
2. Thyrotoxicosis	Atrial fibrillation
3. Rheumatic heart disease	Atrial fibrillation
4. Previous myocardial infarction	Ventricular tachycardia
5. Monoamine oxidase inhibitors (+ tyramin- containing food)	Sinus tachycardia
Bronchodilators	Sinus tachycardia, atrial or ventricular tachycardia
Beta-blockers	Bradycardia (usually sinus)
Tricyclic anti- depressants	Atrial tachycardia

Table 6.3 Symptoms of arrhythmias

Palpitations
Dizziness/syncope
Chest pain
Dyspnea
Sweating
Nausea

which immediately suggest heart disease as the underlying cause. For example, dizziness, which may be produced by either tachycardia or bradycardia (Table 6.3).

(2) Some patients find it difficult to describe the sensation caused by an arrhythmia and may simply complain of feeling 'odd'.

(3) Patients do not necessarily attach the same meaning to words as doctors do. It is, therefore, important always to ask what is meant by, for example, 'palpitations'.

(4) Patients vary in their awareness of alterations in the heart's action. Some are alarmed by what is no more than a moderate sinus tachycardia while others virtually ignore extremely rapid rates: the patient's subjective response to an arrhythmia tells us very little about it.

The objectives, when assessing a patient with a suspected arrhythmia, are as follows:

(1) To determine the nature of the arrhythmia and thus the urgency of, or need for, treatment.
(2) To discover any underlying cause.
(3) To assess the effects of the arrhythmia on the patient's way of life, i.e. the inconvenience caused by it.

The patient should be asked about the frequency and duration of attacks, whether the onset and termination of an attack is sudden or gradual, any precipitant and current drug therapy.

Specific points to look for on examination include evidence of valvular hypertensive heart disease and cardiac failure. The patient's thyroid status should be assessed. Occult infection (such as bronchopneumonia in the elderly) or blood loss may account for an otherwise unexplained sinus tachycardia.

Rational treatment depends on accurate diagnosis and this requires an electrocardiogram recorded during an attack. Family doctors equipped with an electrocardiograph are in the best position to do this, because frequently, by the time a patient arrives at hospital the attack is over. When it proves impossible to record an ECG during an attack, as is often the case, a 24-hour ECG tape monitor can be used. This consists of a small pocket-sized tape recorder which records the ECG continuously for a period of 24 hours or which can be activated by the patient at the onset of an attack.

SUPRAVENTRICULAR TACHYCARDIAS

Sinus tachycardia

Sinus tachycardia is not an arrhythmia in the same sense as the other arrhythmias which will be discussed in this chapter because, although the rapid beating of the heart may cause unpleasant palpitations, sinus tachycardia occurs only as a response to physiological, psychological or pathological stress (see Table 6.4). Therefore, treatment should be directed towards alleviating the underlying condition. There is rarely justification for giving drugs whose only action is to slow the heart rate.

Table 6.4   Common causes of sinus tachycardia

1. Physiological
   Exercise
   Anxiety

2. Pathological
   Pyrexia
   Cardiac failure
   Pain
   Anemia
   Thyrotoxicosis

Paroxysmal atrial tachycardia

This is characterized by a rapid, usually regular heart rate of 160 to 220 beats per minute (Figure 6.1). The attack begins and ends suddenly – an important point to elicit from the history. An attack may last for anything from a few minutes to several days. In some patients attacks occur daily while others may have only one or two attacks per year. Women are more often affected than men. In most cases, no serious underlying pathology is found. The electrocardiogram recorded during an attack shows rapidly recurring, usually normal, QRS complexes. The P wave, which, when visible, tends to be slightly abnormal, may be hidden in the preceding T wave.

Children rarely have paroxysmal tachycardia but when they do it

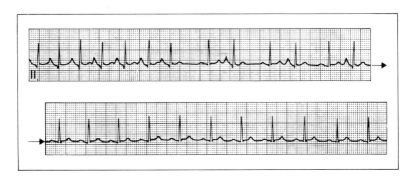

Figure 6.1 Paroxysmal atrial tachycardia. At the beginning of this long record of lead II the QRS complexes are normal and occur regularly at a rate of 136 per minute. After the seventh complex the patient reverts to sinus rhythm but with coupled atrial extrasystoles. The bottom strip shows regular normal sinus rhythm

is usually of this type. The heart rate, especially in infants, may be extremely rapid – up to 300 beats per minute or more.

A number of patients with a supraventricular tachycardia will have an abnormal ECG between attacks. The abnormality consists of a short P–R interval and a slurred QRS complex. This is the Wolff-Parkinson-White syndrome (Figure 6.2) and 70% of patients with this condition suffer from at least one episode of paroxysmal tachycardia during their lifetime. Some patients have distressingly frequent prolonged attacks of tachycardia, often with ventricular rates of over 200 beats per minute.

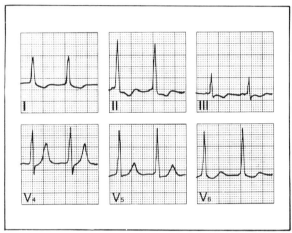

Figure 6.2   The Wolff–Parkinson–White syndrome. The PR interval is short (best seen in lead II), the QRS complexes are abnormally broad and at the beginning of the QRS there is a slurred upstroke, a delta wave (best seen in leads II, V_5 and V_6)

Treatment

An acute attack may be terminated by vagal stimulation, induced by the Valsalva maneuver, eyeball pressure, gagging or carotid sinus massage (Figure 6.3).

Drug treatment may include an intravenous injection of verapamil 5 to 10 mg, or of a beta-blocker (e.g. practolol 10 to 20 mg) which will terminate most attacks. It is important to remember that verapamil *must not* be given within six hours of a beta-blocker as the combination may produce a profound bradycardia. Other

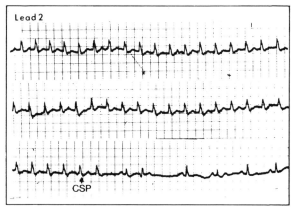

Figure 6.3 Supraventricular tachycardia. The attack is terminated by carotid sinus pressure (CSP)

drugs which may be used include digoxin, procainamide, quinidine and disopryamide. The same drugs are used singly or in various combinations for prophylaxis.

Not all patients require either drug treatment or prophylaxis. Short-lived infrequent attacks are best treated by reassurance.

Resistant cases should be transferred to hospital where DC cardioversion (which is almost always effective) is available. The indications for hospitalization are shown in Table 6.5.

Table 6.5 Indications for hospitalization in patients with paroxysmal atrial tachycardia

1. Shock (cold, clammy, hypotensive)
2. Prolonged attack
3. Chest pain
4. Cardiac failure

Atrial flutter

Atrial flutter usually produces a regular pulse rate of 130 to 170 beats per minute for, although the atrial rate is 260 to 340 beats per minute, only every second impulse gets through to the ventricles. There is usually significant underlying heart disease. Rheumatic heart disease and thyrotoxicosis are the commonest etiologies, but ischemic heart disease and hypertension are responsible for a

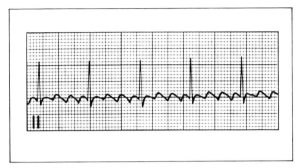

Figure 6.4 Atrial flutter. There are regular symmetrical F (flutter) waves in lead II with no isolectric interval. The QRS complexes are also regular but at a slower rate. This is atrial flutter with 4:1 atrioventricular block

number of cases. The electrocardiogram shows a pathognomonic 'saw-toothed' appearance due to the 'flutter waves' (Figure 6.4). The response to carotid sinus massage is also characteristic; it produces a sudden temporary halving of the pulse rate.

Treatment

Digitalization, possibly with the addition of a beta-blocker, will control the ventricular rate at rest but troublesome tachycardias may still occur at times of exertion or excitement. Sinus rhythm can be restored by a DC shock but very often atrial flutter will recur. This drug treatment is preferable for chronic atrial flutter.

Atrial fibrillation

Atrial fibrillation is the best known pathological arrhythmia (Figure 6.5). It produces an irregularly irregular heart rate of usually well over 100 beats per minute. The radial pulse rate may be slower than this as many of the beats are so weak that the pulse cannot be felt at the wrist. Underlying heart disease is usually present, although this may be difficult to detect because of the rapid heart rate. Rheumatic mitral valve disease is the commonest cause, followed by thyrotoxicosis, ischemic and hypertensive heart disease. Atrial fibrillation, paroxysmal or sustained, without any

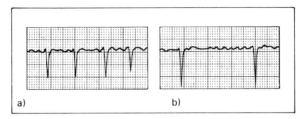

Figure 6.5   Atrial fibrillation. The base line shows fast irregular undulation from the fibrillating atria. In a) the ventricular rate is fast and irregular. In b), which is recorded from the same patient after digitalis has been given, the fast irregular base line fluctuation persists, indicating atrial fibrillation as before but the ventricular rate has been slowed

detectable cardiac lesion is labelled 'lone atrial fibrillation' and is particularly common in middle-aged men.

The arrhythmia may initially be paroxysmal in patients with mitral valve disease but later it becomes established. Atrial fibrillation is poorly tolerated by patients with rheumatic heart disease. It often causes cardiac failure which cannot be controlled until the heart rate is slowed.

Treatment

Digitalization is usually effective in controlling the ventricular rate although, as with atrial flutter, the addition of a beta-blocker may be needed to achieve this. Some patients with 'lone' atrial fibrillation (see above) and selected patients with mitral valve disease are candidates for cardioversion. Those with mitral valve disease, whether the arrhythmia is sustained or paroxysmal, require long-term anticoagulants to reduce the risk of systemic emboli. As noted previously, specialist advice should be sought if the cause cannot be found.

VENTRICULAR TACHYCARDIA

Ventricular tachycardia has the most sinister reputation of all the arrhythmias considered here. There are two reasons for this:

(1) It may progress to ventricular fibrillation.

(2) Because of its association with severe ischemic heart disease
     it is poorly tolerated. If it remains untreated, cardiac failure
     or shock rapidly supervene.

The electrocardiographic diagnosis of ventricular tachycardia is
based on the finding of rapid (120 to 160 beats per minute), more or
less regular, wide QRS complexes interspersed with occasional
normal beats (Figure 6.6).

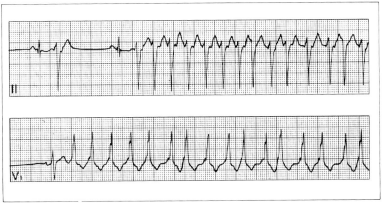

Figure 6.6   Ventricular tachycardia. The first sinus beat is followed by a ventricular
extrasystole. The next beat is sinus and thereafter there is a rapid tachycardia. The
QRS complexes are of the same configuration as the ventricular extrasystole and this
is a run of ventricular tachycardia. Lead V_1 shows the same situation – one normal
sinus beat followed by a burst of ventricular tachycardia

Treatment

Because of its serious nature, all patients with suspected ventricular
tachycardia should be hospitalized. A bolus injection of lignocaine
100 mg intravenously is given over a two minute period and
repeated in 10 minutes if necessary. In many cases this will abolish
the existing attack. Hospital treatment, in the absence of a prompt
response to lignocaine, consists of DC cardioversion followed by
an infusion of lignocaine at a rate of 3 mg per minute for 24 to 36
hours. Several drugs have proved useful for long-term prophylaxis:
procainamide, quinidine, disopyramide, mexiletine and the beta-
blockers.

BRADYCARDIA

The causes of bradycardia are listed in Table 6.6.

Table 6.6   Causes of bradycardia

1. Sinus bradycardia
   a) Physiological (athletes, vasovagal attack)
   b) Drugs – beta-blockers, digoxin
   c) Sick sinus syndrome
   d) Myxedema
2. Heart block
   a) Degenerative fibrosis
   b) Myocardial infarction
   c) Congenital (rare)
   d) Infection, trauma, drugs

Sinus bradycardia

This is the term applied to a normal heart rhythm with a rate of less than 60 beats per minute (Figure 6.7). It requires no treatment in the absence of symptoms. However, care should be taken not to overlook the occasional patient in whom sinus bradycardia is a feature of some other condition, such as myxedema, hypopituitarism, jaundice or raised intracranial pressure. Furthermore, in some patients an apparent sinus bradycardia may prove, on further investigation, to be caused by sino-atrial block (in which profound bradycardia is caused by the omission of complete cardiac cycles) or to be the presenting feature of the 'sick sinus' syndrome. These conditions may require long-term cardiac pacing.

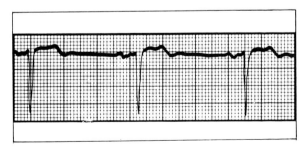

Figure 6.7   Sinus bradycardia, rate 47 per minute. Each PQRST complex is normal

Heart block (atrioventricular block)

When impulses from the sino-atrial node are prevented from reaching the ventricle, heart block is said to exist. When this occurs the ventricles contract at their own rate of less than 40 beats per minute (Figure 6.8). The usual cause of heart block is degenerative fibrosis of part of the conducting system, a process which progresses with age. Sometimes it is caused by myocardial infarction and, rarely, it occurs as a congenital lesion.

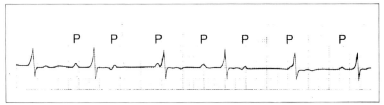

Figure 6.8 Complete heart block, with the ventricular pacemaker situated low down in the ventricles. This type of pacemaker is slow and unreliable. The P waves are regular but the PR interval is completely variable. The QRS complexes, which are abnormally broad, also occur regularly at a rate slower than the P waves

By itself, the slow heart rate produced by heart block is often symptomless. However, many patients (approximately two-thirds) complain of dizziness and others have frank syncope (Stokes–Adams attacks). The latter are caused by transient asystole or, paradoxically, a rapid ventricular arrhythmia. Because death may occur during such an attack, a permanent pacemaker is indicated for all symptomatic patients with heart block. It is difficult to predict who will develop symptoms and therefore all patients with heart block should be considered for permanent pacing. It has been estimated that approximately 50 new cases of heart block per million population occur each year and that now, one hundred pacemakers are implanted annually per million population.

Technique of pacemaker implantation

In most UK centers, pacemakers are implanted in the upper anterior chest wall. The electrode which stimulates the heart is passed to the apex of the right ventricle, under X-ray control, via the subclavian or cephalic vein. The procedure, which usually takes half to one hour, is performed under local anesthetic. The patient can be discharged from hospital 48 to 72 hours postoperatively. The stitches should be removed a week later. The functioning of the pacemaker is tested in the pacemaker clinic after two to four weeks and then at six- to twelve-monthly intervals. The present range of pacemakers is highly reliable and each has a projected 'life' of seven to twelve years or more. Figure 6.9 shows the normal paced ECG.

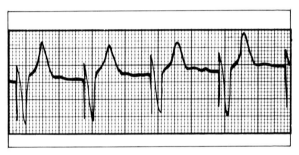

Figure 6.9   Paced ECG. Pacing 'spikes' are followed by wide QRS complexes. This example is taken from a patient with a permanent pacemaker

Most family doctors have no more than one or two patients with pacemakers in their practice, and will consequently have little experience of the occasional problems which occur. The following points should be remembered:

(1) Premature electronic failure of pacemakers is rare. Occasionally, however, during the early weeks after implantation, the tip of the pacing electrode becomes displaced. As a result, pacing ceases and the heart rate slows. If at any time the patient's pulse rate is significantly less than that of the pacemaker (usually 70 beats per minute) specialist advice should be sought.

(2) The pacemaker only prevents bradycardia. Some patients develop tachycardia which does not necessarily mean that the pacemaker is faulty.

(3) The modern range of pacemakers is unaffected by household electrical devices.

(4) Very occasionally the implantation site becomes infected soon after the operation. If this happens the patient should be referred to the local pacemaker clinic.

DRUG-INDUCED ARRHYTHMIAS

It is not surprising that, with the vast range of drugs available to use, some will adversely affect the cardiac rhythm. Drugs affecting the heart rhythm are not always those used to treat heart disease.

Digoxin

It has been estimated that more than 20% of patients taking digoxin experience side-effects at some time. The most important factors which predispose to digoxin toxicity are old age, hypokalemia and renal failure. As many older digitalized patients are also on diuretic therapy, diuretic-induced hypokalemia can occur, in which case a potassium-sparing diuretic may be used, such as triamterene. Digoxin may produce a wide variety of arrhythmias.

Bradycardia. Too much digoxin classically causes bradycardia. The rhythm may be sinus bradycardia, sino-atrial block or heart block. A pulse rate below 60 beats per minute suggests the possibility of toxicity.

Ectopic beats. Second to bradycardia, ventricular ectopic beats are the best known manifestation of digoxin toxicity. These may take several forms:

(1) Infrequent ventricular extrasystoles.
(2) One ectopic beat coupled with each normal beat causing a bigeminal rhythm (Figure 6.10).
(3) Multifocal ventricular extrasystoles, i.e. ectopic beats with different shapes on the electrocardiogram.
(4) Short runs of ventricular tachycardia.

Although digoxin toxicity typically causes bradycardia or ventricular ectopics it is important to remember that it sometimes causes

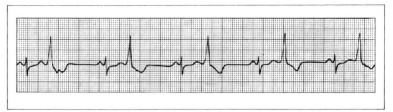

Figure 6.10 Excessive dosage of digitalis causing coupled ventricular extrasystoles. The tracing shows sinus rhythm but every second beat is wide and bizarre and is followed by a compensatory pause

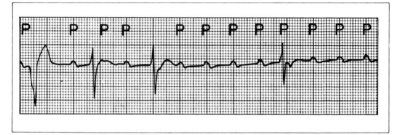

Figure 6.11 Paroxysmal atrial tachycardia with block as a result of excessive digitalis medication. Regular P waves occur at a rate of 1150 per minute and the QRS complexes occur irregularly. The regular P waves are best seen when the ventricular rate is slow

tachycardia. Atrial tachycardia with block (Figure 6.11) and accelerated nodal tachycardia are particularly suggestive of over-dosage – indeed every known type of tachycardia has, on occasion, been attributed to digoxin toxicity. The practical implication of this is that it should not be assumed, as it often is, that an increase in pulse rate in a digitalized patient calls for more digoxin – the reverse may be the case.

If toxicity is suspected, digoxin should be withdrawn and the blood levels of potassium and urea estimated to discover whether uremia or hypokalemia is a predisposing factor.

Procainamide and quinidine

These two drugs, which are used to treat ventricular arrhythmias, may themselves increase ventricular excitability and cause ventricular ectopics, ventricular tachycardia or even ventricular fibrillation.

Sympathomimetic amines

Drugs of this group, such as isoprenaline and ephedrine, are commonly used to treat bronchospasm. Sinus tachycardia occurs frequently during treatment and may cause unpleasant palpitations. Ventricular ectopic beats, ventricular tachycardia and ventricular fibrillation have caused death in some cases.

Tricyclic antidepressants

Sinus tachycardia is common, due to the atropine-like effects of this group of drugs, and ventricular arrhythmias are occasionally seen. The risk of sudden death is slightly increased in patients with heart disease who are being treated with the tricyclic antidepressants but this risk is so small that in most cases there should be no hesitation in giving a tricyclic antidepressant when the psychiatric state is one of severe depression.

Phenothiazines

This group of tranquilizers includes chlorpromazine and thioridazine. Ventricular arrhythmias have occasionally been reported with therapeutic dosages.

7
Myocardial Infarction

C. WARD and J. FLEMING

Coronary artery disease is the commonest cause of death in men over the age of 45 years in the western world. In the UK, 30% of all male deaths in the 35 to 45 year age-group are caused by coronary artery disease and the figure is even higher amongst those aged between 45 and 55 years. 50 to 60% of such deaths occur suddenly. This has been discussed in detail in Chapter 1. However, the major risk factors bear repeating because their correction, when possible, offers the best prospect of reducing the incidence of coronary disease.

RISK FACTORS

(1) *Cigarette smoking*. A man who smokes 20 cigarettes per day has at least a ten-fold increased risk of dying from coronary disease compared with a non-smoker.

(2) Hypertension. The incidence of myocardial infarction is almost linearly related to both systolic and diastolic blood pressure. This applies to any level above 140/90 mmHg which many doctors do not regard as abnormal and do not treat.

(3) *Hypercholesterolemia*. A serum cholesterol of 300 mg % or more is associated with a three- to four-fold increased risk of myocardial infarction compared with values below 200 mg %.

(4) *Others*. Other important risk factors include a family

history of coronary artery disease, increasing age and the male sex. Diabetes mellitus carries a high risk of myocardial infarction with an especially high mortality. The influence of physical inactivity, mental stress, obesity and hyperuricemia is less clearly defined.

PRESENTATION

The reduction of coronary blood flow to a point where myocardial necrosis occurs produces acute myocardial infarction. In the majority of cases this gives rise to characteristic clinical features.

The typical prolonged retrosternal pain is variously described as 'crushing', 'vice-like' or 'gripping'. Often there is a history of angina which has increased in severity and frequency prior to the attack. Diagnostic difficulties may occur as follows:

(1) The pain may be of relatively short duration. In general terms, cardiac pain which lasts for less than 15 minutes is unlikely to be associated with infarction, whereas, when the duration of pain is greater than half an hour, it often is. Pain of intermediate duration, i.e. of 15 to 30 minutes duration, is very much a diagnostic 'grey area'.

(2) The pain is occasionally confined exclusively to one of the sites to which cardiac pain often radiates – the neck, jaw, shoulder or arm.

(3) The patient may present with acute left ventricular failure and the associated distress may mask concurrent chest discomfort.

(4) Myocardial infarction can be painless, particularly in the elderly.

The chest pain of myocardial infarction is frequently accompanied by nausea, vomiting, faintness, sweating or palpitations.

FINDINGS ON EXAMINATION

The aims of the examination are to detect the presence and extent of hemodynamic impairment caused by the suspected infarction.

(1) *Blood pressure.* Initially, the blood pressure is usually normal or moderately elevated. Within 24 hours the level falls as a result of the infarction. Severe hypotension at the onset, when associated with a low cardiac output, is a grave sign usually indicating cardiogenic shock.

(2) *Heart rate and rhythm.* Sinus tachycardia is common as a result of pain, anxiety or cardiac failure. Some patients have a sinus bradycardia, especially when the infarction affects the inferior wall: increased vagal tone is usually responsible. In other cases, bradycardia is a result of heart block.

(3) *Auscultation.* The heart sounds are softer than usual, with a fourth heart sound frequently audible. A third sound suggests cardiac failure and is less common. Occasionally a loud systolic murmur appears in the early days after infarction, indicating rupture of the interventricular septum or of a papillary muscle. This is accompanied by severe cardiac failure. Less obvious, transient mitral murmurs are common and indicate temporary impairment of papillary muscle function. A faint pericardial rub from localized pericarditis is sometimes heard. In 15% of cases a loud rub appears after the third day and this indicates generalized pericarditis.

Auscultation of the chest may reveal fine basal crepitations due to pulmonary edema, but a chest X-ray is a more accurate method of detecting lung congestion.

DIAGNOSIS

The diagnosis of acute myocardial infarction is based on the history aided by the electrocardiogram. Enzyme tests are used to confirm the diagnosis or, quantitatively, to indicate the extent of myocardial damage.

(1) *Pain.* Patients with a typical history of prolonged cardiac pain can almost invariably be shown to have had an acute myocardial infarction. Many intra-abdominal and intrathoracic pathologies are listed in the differential diagnosis of myocardial infarction but when the history is

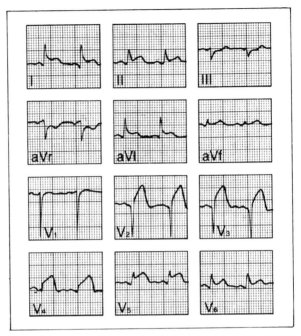

Figure 7.1 Pathological Q waves appear in leads V_2, V_3 and V_4. This indicates a diagnosis of myocardial infarction

taken carefully, confusion with other conditions is not common.

(2) *Electrocardiogram.* The characteristic features of myocardial infarction which appear on the ECG are (a) pathological Q waves (Figure 7.1), (b) ST segment elevation with an upward convexity (Figure 7.2) and (c) T wave inversion (Figure 7.3). The changes indicate necrosis, injury and ischemia respectively. Over the course of a few weeks or months the ST segment and T wave changes often revert, but Q waves are more persistent. If ST segment elevation is still present after six months, a ventricular aneurysm should be suspected (Figure 7.4).

The leads in which ECG changes occur indicate the site of infarction and are as follows: Leads I, aVl, V_5 and V_6 – anterolateral (Figure 7.5); leads II, III and aVf – inferior (Figure 7.6); leads V_2 to V_4 – septal.

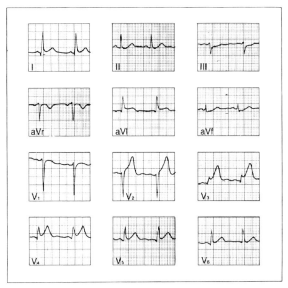

Figure 7.2   There is definite ST segment elevation in leads I, aVl, V₂, V₃ and V₅. The patient showed clinical features of myocardial infarction, and this would be a probable diagnosis on the electrocardiogram. There are no Q waves, however, and the diagnosis could not be made with great confidence from this electrocardiogram alone

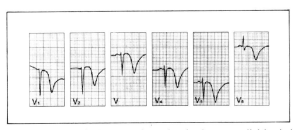

Figure 7.3   Deep symmetrical T wave inversion in the precordial leads is shown. The shape of these T waves makes the diagnosis of myocardial infarction probable, and this was the diagnosis in this patient

(3) *Enzymes.* Cellular death results in the release of the enzymes normally contained within cells. When this happens to a large number of cells, as in acute myocardial infarction, sufficient quantities of the enzymes are released into the circulation for them to be detectable in the serum. The most

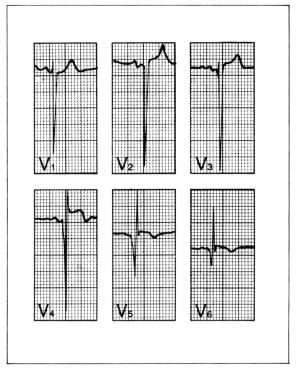

Figure 7.4   Q waves are present in leads V_4, V_5 and V_6, the ST segment is elevated in those leads and the T wave is inverted. Recent anterolateral myocardial infarction is a possible diagnosis but the history indicates that an infarction occurred six months previously and that many ECGs over a period of some months have shown persistent ST segment elevation. The diagnosis of left ventricular aneurysm following myocardial infarction was made, and the aneurysm resected at operation with considerable improvement in the patient's signs and symptoms of cardiac failure

commonly used enzyme tests are shown in Table 7.1. Unfortunately, with the possible exception of MB-CPK, these enzymes are not exclusive to heart muscle. Consequently, elevated serum enzyme levels do not necessarily indicate myocardial damage. Thus, when the history and electrocardiogram are atypical, a diagnosis of acute myocardial infarction should not be based upon a modest serum enzyme elevation. The serum levels of most routinely tested enzymes revert to normal after about five days and it is therefore

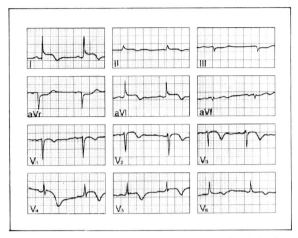

Figure 7.5 Anterolateral myocardial infarction. ST elevation in leads I and aVl with T wave inversion in V_2 to V_6. Note the flat contour of the elevated ST segment

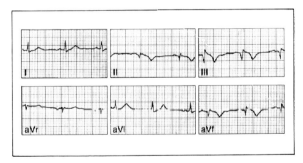

Figure 7.6 Inferior myocardial infarction. Pathological Q waves are present in leads II, III and aVf. The T wave is deeply inverted in these leads

pointless to request enzyme assays if the suspected infarction occurred more than a few days before a blood sample is taken.

GENERAL MANAGEMENT

The principles of management involve adequate rest, relief of pain and anxiety, and appropriate therapy for cardiac failure and arrhythmias.

Table 7.1 Commonly used enzyme tests

Enzyme test	Normal range[1]	Time-scale of elevated levels		
		Onset	Peak	Duration
SGOT (AST)	<15	10 hrs	18 to 36 hrs	3 to 4 days
LHD	<240	24 to 48 hrs	3 to 6 days	10 to 14 days
HBDH	<140	12 to 36 hrs	3 to 6 days	8 to 10 days
CPK (SCK)	<50	6 to 8 hrs	24 hrs	3 to 4 days
MB-CPK	<5	6 to 8 hrs	12 to 24 hrs	1 to 4 days

[1] All measured in U/l at 25 °C. Figures will vary from one laboratory to another

Nowadays, patients with a mild myocardial infarction are kept in bed for only 48 hours. Thereafter, gradual mobilization should ensure that they can gently walk around the room or ward by the end of a week. Even when cardiac failure has been present, it is usually possible to get the patient out of bed after a week or 10 days. Early mobilization not only reduces the incidence of deep vein thrombosis and pulmonary embolism but also probably improves the chances of subsequent full recovery.

A powerful analgesic is usually required for the relief of pain, e.g. morphine 10 to 15 mg or heroin 5 to 10 mg intramuscularly or intravenously. The addition of an antiemitic, such as cyclizine 50 mg, reduces the incidence of vomiting, but does not affect the hypotension and bradycardia which occur in some patients.

Many patients are understandably anxious and although reassurance helps, it is often advisable to give a mild tranquilizer, such as diazepam 2 to 5 mg t.i.d.

There is no evidence that oxygen is of value in uncomplicated cases but the arterial PO_2 is always below normal and oxygen should certainly be given whenever cardiac failure is present.

Evidence of a beneficial effect from anticoagulant therapy is conflicting. A reasonable compromise, adopted by many coronary care units, is to give either warfarin or subcutaneous heparin to patients while they are immobilized, except when there is evidence of pericarditis.

Complications and their treatment

The majority of early complications, i.e. those occurring within a week or 10 days of the infarction, can be grouped under two headings:

(1) Arrhythmias, most of which are related to electrical instability of ischemic myocardium or to injury to part of the conducting tissue.
(2) Mechanical impairment of function resulting from destruction of or injury to large areas of myocardium.

Arrhythmias

Ventricular arrhythmias. Ventricular arrhythmias of all types are especially common in the early hours after the onset of myocardial infarction and the incidence falls rapidly after about six hours.

Ventricular ectopic beats occur in virtually all patients with acute myocardial infarction. Treatment to suppress the ectopic beats is usually recommended if they are very frequent, if they are multifocal or if they occur on the T wave of the preceding beat. Lignocaine is usually the drug of first choice and is given as 100 to 150 mg intravenous bolus followed by an infusion to 2 to 5 mg/minute for 24 to 48 hours. Effective alternatives are practolol, procainamide, disopyramide and mexiletine.

Ventricular tachycardia occurs in 5 to 10% of patients. It causes a profound fall in cardiac output and, if untreated, is followed by ventricular fibrillation. If a bolus of lignocaine does not rapidly restore sinus rhythm, DC cardioversion must be used.

Ventricular fibrillation occurs in approximately 10% of patients in coronary care units and requires immediate direct current shock. This is usually administered by the nurse in charge, as prompt action is vital.

Bradycardia. Sinus bradycardia occurs in more than 30% of patients. It is usually transient and of no consequence. However, more profound bradycardia may be accompanied by hypotension or cardiac failure. Elevation of the foot of the bed may be all that is needed to increase the heart rate. In other cases, atropine 0.6 to 1.2 mg i.v. has to be given, sometimes repeatedly.

Heart block. Either second degree (Figure 7.7) or complete heart block occurs in more than 5% of cases. Atropine is often ineffective and in most coronary care units a temporary endo-cardial pacemaker is used to ensure that an adequate heart rate is maintained.

Other arrhythmias. Atrial tachycardia, atrial flutter and atrial fibrillation are all seen occasionally. The associated rapid ventricular rate is poorly tolerated. Digoxin, alone or with a beta-blocker will adequately control the heart rate in most cases, but if this combination fails, DC cardioversion should be used.

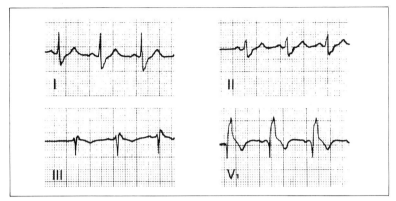

Figure 7.7 This patient presented with chest pain. QRS is 0.12 seconds in duration. There is terminal R^1 wave in lead V_1: indicating complete right bundle branch block. This was caused by involvement of the right bundle branch by a myocardial infarction

Complications caused by impaired function or mechanical defect

These include cardiac failure, cardiogenic shock, cardiac rupture, papillary muscle rupture, ventricular septal defect and ventricular aneurysm.

(1) *Cardiac failure.* Evidence of left ventricular failure can be detected in more than two-thirds of patients with myocardial infarction. It is usually mild and the diagnosis is based on the finding of one or more of the expected clinical features – sinus tachycardia, gallop rhythm and basal crepitations. In other cases typical acute pulmonary edema occurs. In the mild cases only a diuretic is needed but when the condition is more severe, digoxin should be included in the treatment. All cases should be treated with continuous oxygen.

(2) *Cardiogenic shock.* Approximately 10% of patients with acute myocardial infarction develop features of shock, i.e. hypotension, poor tissue perfusion (cold, clammy extremities) and oliguria (urine flow of less than 30 ml/hr.) Postmortem studies have shown that shock is usually associated with extensive myocardial infarction. The mortality is approximately 90%. The use of vasodilators,

such as intravenous nitroprusside may help but requires careful hemodynamic monitoring.

Circulatory assistance with the intra-aortic balloon pump may help the patient over the first few days but this form of treatment is only available in specialist cardiology centers and its usefulness is controversial.

(3) *Cardiac rupture* is responsible for 5 to 10% of deaths from acute myocardial infarction. It occurs within the first few days after infarction and causes sudden death.

(4) *Rupture of a papillary muscle* or of the interventricular septum occurs in approximately 2% of cases. Each event usually precipitates cardiogenic shock and is associated with a harsh systolic murmur. The mortality is very high but patients may be saved by intensive circulatory support followed by appropriate surgery.

(5) *Ventricular aneurysm* (Figure 7.8) develops in about 20% of cases. Many are not recognized clinically. The diagnosis should be suspected in the following situations: persistent cardiac failure, recurrent ventricular arrhythmias or systemic emboli.

Suspicion may be strengthened by the finding of a para-doxical pulsation above or medial to the apex beat. In these patients cardiac catheterization is indicated to define the extent of the aneurysm and associated coronary artery disease. The presence of an aneurysm may not be suspected until weeks or months after the infarction occurs.

(6) *Other complications.* Pericarditis occurs in at least 10% of cases. Characteristically, the patient complains of pleuro-pericardial pain between the third day after infarction and the end of the first week. An accompanying pericardial rub is usually audible for two to three days. These patients must not be given anticoagulant therapy as this may cause hemo-pericardium.

Pulmonary emboli are relatively uncommon now that early mobilization is widely practised. Systemic emboli sometimes occur and usually arise from thrombus formed in the left ventricle at the site of infarction.

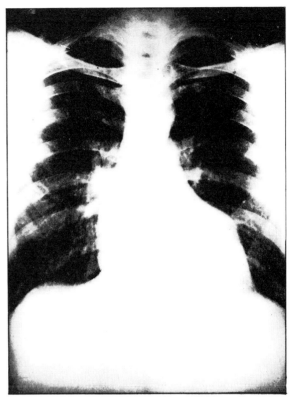

Figure 7.8   Chest radiograph showing a slightly enlarged cardiac shadow (cardiac ratio 16/32). An abnormal bulge is visible on the left heart border. The appearance suggests ventricular aneurysm. Cardiac catheterization is indicated in order to confirm the diagnosis

Late complications

Late complications of myocardial infarction include angina, cardiac failure, reinfarction, sudden death and post myocardial infarction syndrome.

Angina develops in up to 50% of patients following myocardial infarction. Treatment with trinitrin should constitute the initial management, and a beta-blocker may be added if necessary. Coronary artery surgery is considered if the angina interferes with the patient's lifestyle. Persistent cardiac failure usually indicates that myocardial damage has been extensive. In some it is associated with a respectable ventricular aneurysm, but this can only be established by angiocardiography. If no surgically correctable lesion is found, treatment for the cardiac failure should be along the usual lines of rest, diuretics and digitalization.

In general terms, the incidence of reinfarction during the first two years after myocardial infarction is approximately 10% and the incidence of sudden death during the same period is somewhat higher.

The post myocardial infarction syndrome affects a small percentage of patients. Symptoms, which begin one to six weeks after infarction, consist of pleuropericardial pain (often with a friction rub) and pyrexia. Most patients recover within a few days. When symptoms are severe or prolonged, steroids are dramatically effective.

PROGNOSIS

Numerous factors influence the prognosis following acute myocardial infarction. Several of these are clearly related to the extent of the infarction and the degree of coronary atheroma. Left ventricular failure, cardiomegaly, bundle branch block, previous infarction and recurrent arrhythmias all worsen the outlook. Other adverse factors are age, hypertension and diabetes mellitus.

It must also be remembered that 50 to 60% of deaths from acute myocardial infarction occur during the first six hours, so that survival rates quoted by coronary care units will depend upon the speed with which patients are transferred to hospital (Figure 7.9). Bearing in mind all of these variable and often interrelated factors, the overall hospital mortality is about 15 to 20%.

Following discharge from hospital, the prognosis is likewise mainly determined by the extent of the infarction. The other factors mentioned also play a part, as does continuation of cigarette smoking. In general terms, the mortality rate during the first year is approximately 15%. Thereafter, the annual mortality is 3 to 4% and the 10-year survival rate is around 60%. More specifically, the annual mortality following myocardial infarction has been related to the number of diseased vessels assessed at coronary angio-

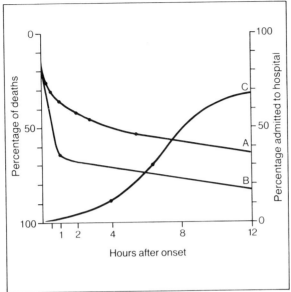

Figure 7.9 Graph of deaths following myocardial infarction plotted against time. A = All age-groups of patients admitted to hospital. B = Males under 50 years of age. C = Admission time following infarction. (Courtesy of H. Baird.)

graphy, thus one diseased vessel has a mortality rate of 1 to 2%, two vessels 4 to 5%, three vessels 9 to 10%, and left main stem 15 to 20%.

REHABILITATION

There is an understandable tendency for patients to become intro-spective following a myocardial infarction. This is unfortunately often reinforced by the well-intentioned advice from relatives and doctors 'not to overdo things'. The psychological effects of this are a major factor in the delayed return to work and to a normal life-style which is so common following a myocardial infarction.

From early convalescence, the patient and near relatives should be encouraged that a return to normal physical activity within a matter of a few weeks is not only possible, but also safe and beneficial. The question of sexual problems is rarely broached by either patient or doctor. This causes much unnecessary mental anguish both to patient and spouse. The patient should be advised that in most cases normal sexual activity can be safely resumed within a few weeks.

Within this more positive approach, about half of all patients can return to work within three months and most of the remainder within five to six months. Indeed, most patients whose myocardial infarction was uncomplicated and whose work does not involve heavy lifting can return to full employment in eight weeks or less. However, patients whose work involves long-distance driving are the exception and even social driving should be discouraged for about two months. A history of myocardial infarction is a contraindication to holding a Heavy Goods Vehicle Licence, and Public Service Vehicle Licences are likewise usually withdrawn. The patient should be advised to inform his employer about the nature of his illness.

CONVALESCENT ASSESSMENT

Family doctors and hospital consultants alike foster the patient's tendency to introspection by insisting on too frequent visits to the surgery or outpatient clinic. Nevertheless, it is important that all patients should be carefully examined approximately three months after infarction (Table 7.2). This examination should have the following objectives:

Table 7.2   The three-month post-infarction examination

1. Look for evidence of:
   Cardiac failure
   Ventricular aneurysm
   Arrhythmias

2. Assess:
   Severity of angina
   Blood pressure
   Functional capacity

3. Take blood for:
   Lipids
   Glucose

4. Advise against smoking

(1) To assess the after-effects of the myocardial infarction and to determine the need for treatment of any complications.

(2) To discover the presence of risk factors, correction of which may improve the prognosis. With this in mind, the following points should be noted:

    (a) Blood pressure. In hypertensive patients, the blood pressure tends to fall following myocardial infarction and only reaches the previous level after several months. There is now evidence that control of the blood pressure with appropriate drugs may reduce the incidence of reinfarction. Thus the three months post-infarction examination is an appropriate time to assess the need for hypotensive therapy.

    (b) Cigarette smoking. There is clear-cut evidence that cessation of smoking reduces the incidence of post-infarction complications. Two years after infarction, the cumulative mortality of former smokers is half that of those who continue to smoke. The reinfarction rate is also halved. Every effort should be made to encourage the patient to give up cigarettes.

    (c) Serum lipids and blood glucose. The blood sugar and lipid patterns are often transiently abnormal during the course of acute myocardial infarction, but any abnormality detected at three months will be signifi cant. The detection of a lipid abnormality – at least in younger patients – warrants treatment. The discovery of diabetes mellitus at any age calls for appropriate therapy.

PREVENTION OF SUDDEN DEATH

Sudden death during the first few months after infarction is a major problem and numerous studies have been and are being conducted to discover whether the incidence can be reduced. Several drugs have been investigated, including clofibrate, the beta-blockers, sulphinpyrazone and aspirin. There is so far no unequivocal evidence that the routine use of any of these drugs is beneficial.

8
Congenital Cardiac Disease

J. FLEMING and C. WARD

The majority of patients with significant congenital heart disease are diagnosed in infancy or childhood. A few escape detection until adult life when, for example, rib notching on a pre-employment chest X-ray reveals the presence of an unsuspected coarctation of the aorta.

PRESENTATION

Cyanosis

The presence of cyanosis in infancy is always significant and, when lung disease can be excluded, implies serious heart disease. The age at which cyanosis appears may be of some diagnostic help. For example, cyanosis detected soon after birth suggests the possibility of tranposition of the great arteries, whereas the child over one year of age who develops cyanosis probably has Fallot's tetralogy. There are, of course, other congenital heart lesions which produce cyanosis, including tricuspid atresia, total anomalous pulmonary venous drainage and truncus arteriosus, but the important point to note is that cyanosis demands urgent investigation.

Cardiac murmurs

A cardiac murmur is often the first indication of heart disease.

Many normal infants and children, however, have quite loud systolic murmurs and a life-threatening congenital cardiac malformation may be present without any detectable murmur. The presence of a murmur in a thriving child may well have no particular significance. The absence of a murmur does not exclude life-threatening congenital heart disease, such as transposition of the great vessels, aortic stenosis and the hypoplastic left heart syndrome, in all of which a murmur is frequently absent.

Heart failure

Heart failure in infancy tends to show itself by a fast respiratory rate, failure to take a full feed, perspiration, restlessness and liver enlargement, rather than by peripheral edema. The less severe cases may merely present as infants who fail to gain weight normally.

MANAGEMENT

Surgical treatment, either corrective or palliative, is now feasible for virtually all congenital cardiac defects and this governs the approach to management. Infants who are clearly ill or who do not improve promptly with medical treatment are investigated fully as a matter of urgency. The aim is to define precisely the anatomical defects and their severity and for this purpose cardiac catheterization and angiocardiography are usually required. When a complete diagnosis has been obtained it is possible to plan the form and timing of cardiac surgery.

CONGENITAL DEFECTS

Eight specific defects account for almost 90% of all congenital heart disease (Table 8.1) and these defects will now be described in more detail.

Table 8.1 Incidence of common congenital heart defects (expressed as a percentage of all congenital heart disease)

Defect	Percentage
Ventricular septal defect	30
Atrial septal defect	10
Pulmonary stenosis	10
Persistent ductus arteriosus	10
Tetralogy of Fallot	10
Aortic stenosis	7
Coarctation of the aorta	5
Transposition of the great vessels	5

Transposition of the great vessels

In this condition the great vessels are wrongly connected, the aorta communicating with the right ventricle and the pulmonary artery with the left. Consequently, blue blood from the great veins flows to the right atrium, right ventricle and then to the aorta without passing through the lungs, and oxygenated blood from the lungs can reach the aorta only if there is a persistent ductus or a defect in the atrial or ventricular septum. Affected infants are blue at birth and, untreated, have a very high mortality in the first weeks and months of life.

Treatment

Urgent investigation by angiocardiography (Figure 8.1) is required for these cyanosed infants and when transposition of the great vessels is found an immediate effort is made to improve the oxygenation of the blood delivered to the aorta. This involves the creation of a large hole in the atrial septum to allow good mixing of oxygenated blood from the left atrium with the right atrial blood. The cardiologist performing the angiocardiogram replaces the standard catheter with a balloon catheter. When the tip of the catheter containing the balloon has been manipulated through the foramen ovale into the left atrium the balloon is inflated and the catheter jerked back into the right atrium, thereby rupturing the interatrial septum. Arterial oxygenation improves immediately and most infants then thrive, allowing cardiac surgery to be performed as a planned procedure in a year or two, with very satisfactory

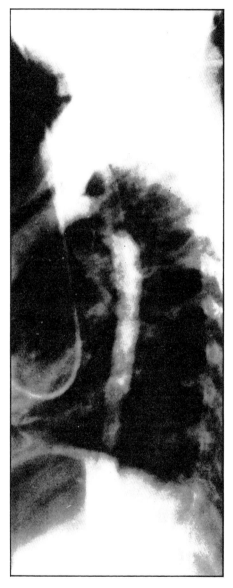

Figure 8.1 Angiogram showing the right ventricle connected to the aorta. The aorta also shows a mild coarctation. This is transposition of the great vessels

results. Many patients initially treated by balloon atrial septostomy and later by extensive cardiac surgery involving the insertion of baffles in the atria to divert blood from the lungs to the aorta are now reaching adulthood and leading active lives. It is too early to ascertain whether surgical correction of transposition can enable patients to achieve a normal lifespan.

The most recent operation involves switching the aorta with the coronary vessels from the right ventricle to the left and reattaching the pulmonary artery to the right ventricle. The operative mortality is higher in this procedure but the long-term prognosis may well be better since the right ventricle is relieved of the burden of maintaining a systemic blood pressure.

Fallot's tetralogy

This is the commonest form of cyanotic congenital heart disease. Those children affected are cyanosed because there is a large ventricular septal defect together with stenosis of the right ventricular outflow tract and this severe infundibular stenosis forces much of the blood in the right ventricle to flow through the defect into the left ventricle and aorta. There is, of course, right ventricular hypertrophy and this, together with over-riding of the aortic root, completes the four abnormalities of Fallot's tetralogy. The more severe is the infundibular stenosis, the earlier and more intense the cyanosis. Often, cyanosis is not detected until the child is nine months old or more. Squatting and attacks of syncope, well known additional symptoms of this condition, are rarely encountered. The symptoms were most characteristic of the older untreated cases.

The diagnosis is suggested by the appearance of cyanosis in a child with a pulmonary systolic murmur, a single second heart sound, right ventricular hypertrophy on the electrocardiogram and poor lung vascular marking on the chest X-ray. Angiocardiography confirms the diagnosis and reveals the extent of the stenosis and the size of the main pulmonary artery. A good surgical result can be expected when the pulmonary artery is reasonably well developed.

Treatment

Correction of Fallot's tetralogy involves surgical closure of the ventricular septal defect together with the removal of the pulmonary infundibular stenosis. This can be accomplished in the first few months of life but the mortality is lower if the operation can be delayed until the child is over one year of age. When the child's condition is poor and it would be dangerous to wait, most centers still perform a temporary shunt operation, such as a Blalock anastomosis of a subclavian artery to the pulmonary artery. This improves the supply of oxygenated blood to the body and allows corrective surgery to be delayed. The disadvantages are that two operations are required and at the second definitive operation there is the complication of closing the Blalock anastomosis.

The surgical results of total correction of Fallot's tetralogy are very good and most patients now survive into adulthood and are able to lead almost normal lives.

Ventricular septal defect

A hole in the septum between the two ventricles is the commonest of all congenital heart defects. Fortunately, in the majority of cases the hole is not large and tends to diminish in size throughout childhood, often resulting in spontaneous closure. In approximately one third of cases the defect forms part of a more complex lesion, such as tetralogy of Fallot.

A loud systolic murmur maximal at the left sternal edge is the commonest mode of presentation, often occurring in an asymptomatic child. The flow of blood is from the high pressure left ventricle to the low pressure right-sided cardiac chambers to the left. There is no central cyanosis. When the diagnosis appears to be that of ventricular septal defect, it is necessary to know the magnitude of the flow through the defect and the pressure in the pulmonary artery. A small flow ventricular septal defect with no pulmonary hypertension does not require cardiac catheterization and cardiac surgery should not be advised.

Treatment

Occasionally a large ventricular septal defect causes heart failure in infancy and surgical closure must be carried out. This operation can now be undertaken with reasonable safety even in early infancy and seems preferable to the old operation of tying a tight band round the pulmonary artery. The band limits the flow of blood to the lungs and initial results were good but a second operation to close the ventricular septal defect was required and carried the additional hazard of removal of the band.

Follow-up at a hospital clinic is recommended for all small ventricular septal defects and at these attendances it must be explained to the parents the desirability of antibiotic administration prior to dental extraction to minimize the possibility of infective endocarditis. There is a small risk of endocarditis in these patients, but the risk is much smaller than that of surgical closure of the defect.

Atrial septal defect

The commonest position for a defect in the atrial septum is in the middle of the septum and this ostium secundum type of defect presents little difficulty in treatment. The less common ostium primum atrial septal defect is situated low down close to the mitral and tricuspid valves and there is always an abnormal mitral valve. When the mitral valve is grossly distorted these patients present a real challenge to the skills of the cardiac surgeon because he must close the atrial septal defect and repair the mitral valve.

Symptoms from an atrial septal defect are unusual in infancy because the full shunt of blood into the lungs does not occur until the initial high pressure in the pulmonary artery has completely subsided. In childhood there tends to be merely a tendency to chest infections with easy tiring. Large atrial septal defects cause the right ventricle to fail in later life and we therefore advise closure of all defects in which the flow of blood to the lungs is greater than twice the systemic flow.

Diagnosis is suggested by the finding of a large heart, a pulmonary systolic murmur and fixed splitting of the second heart sound. A tricuspid diastolic murmur in conjunction with these signs makes the diagnosis more certain. The chest X-ray shows a large heart when the shunt is big and the pulmonary vascular markings are increased because of the large flow of blood through the lungs. The electrocardiogram is helpful, showing some degree of right bundle branch block in most cases, with right axis deviation in the more usual secundum type lesion. Left axis deviation on the electrocardiogram would suggest ostium primum atrial septal defect and left ventricular angiography would then be undertaken as the best means of demonstrating the shape of the left ventricular outflow tract and the condition of the mitral valve.

Persistent ductus arteriosus

Persistence of the ductus arteriosus is very common in premature infants and usually causes little additional trouble, the ductus soon closing spontaneously. Occasionally poor progress and signs of heart failure demand active measures to close the ductus and this may sometimes be achieved by giving indomethacin.

A small persistent ductus in infancy or childhood causes no symptoms and is detected by the presence of a continuous murmur below the left clavicle. A large ductus carries a large shunt from the aorta to the lungs resulting in sharp arterial pulses, cardiac enlargement, and possibly signs of heart failure. The murmur is not always typically continuous and may be only systolic in timing.

Treatment

Surgical closure is the treatment of choice. The morbidity and mortality of this operation are minimal and much less than the dangers of infective endocarditis on the untreated ductus.

Pulmonary valve stenosis

Pulmonary valve stenosis may present as a systolic murmur maximal in the pulmonary area, preceded by a pulmonary ejection click. The chest X-ray shows sparse lung vessel markings and the electrocardiogram shows right ventricular hypertrophy. In this case there would be little difficulty in diagnosis but in infancy the presentation may be simply that of a child in heart failure with a soft systolic murmur and perhaps central cyanosis. The cyanosis is caused by a shunt of blood from right atrium to left atrium through a patent foramen ovale and in this case the pulmonary stenosis is severe.

Treatment

Severe stenosis of the pulmonary valve requires surgical relief. The diagnosis is confirmed by angiocardiography and the severity determined by measuring the pressure difference across the valve during the systole. The cardiac surgeon can usually achieve satis-factory relief of the stenosis by opening the pulmonary artery and carefully incising the deformed pulmonary valve. Surgical relief is necessary even in the asymptomatic patient because severe stenosis leads to increasing right ventricular hypertrophy and fibrosis with inevitable failure in later life.

Coarctation of the aorta

The usual site for narrowing of the aorta lies just distal to the origin of the left subclavian artery. When severe, coarctation is a cause of heart failure in infancy and may be suspected by finding large pulses in the arms and very poor femoral pulses. Rib notching is not seen on the chest X-ray in coarctation until the child reaches the age of seven to nine years.

Treatment

In infancy treatment with digoxin and diuretics may improve the condition of the child so much that surgery can safely be delayed. If there is little improvement, surgery to resect the coarcted segment can be carried out with fairly low risk even in early infancy. The narrowed segment is cut out and the normal aorta joined end to end. Surgical correction is also required in older children and adults for any severe coarctation despite the lack of symptoms. There is an ever-present risk of cerebral hemorrhage, endarteritis, systemic hypertension, heart failure and rupture of the aorta. Results of surgery are good and usually lead to a permanent reduction in blood pressure.

The finding of coarctation in an apparently normal female is much less common than in the male and when coarctation is diagnosed in the female steps should be taken to exclude the chromosome abnormality responsible for Turner's syndrome.

Congenital aortic valve stenosis

In childhood, aortic valve stenosis may be discovered by the finding of a loud murmur at a routine examination in a symptom-free schoolboy. In all cases a very careful assessment of the severity of the stenosis must be undertaken because the absence of symptoms cannot be taken to mean that there is no danger. The first symptom may be sudden death. The cardiologist will assess the severity by clinical examination, electrocardiography, echocardiography, chest X-ray and, if thought necessary, left ventricular angiography (Figure 8.2). A severe stenosis demands surgery at any age but for lesser degrees of severity it should be possible to limit strenuous physical exertion and delay surgery, if possible, until body growth has been fully achieved.

Treatment

Stenosis of the aortic valve can cause trouble at any stage in life. The most severe cases present in infancy with heart failure and require urgent surgery. Quite good results can be obtained despite the severe deformity of the valve cusps usually encountered when surgery proves necessary at this early age. Probably many of these patients will require aortic valve replacement as a second operation when they are older. The initial operation is undertaken to make as adequate an opening as possible through the grossly malformed valve.

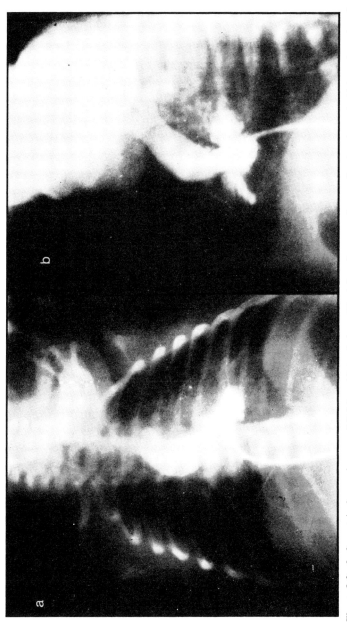

Figure 8.2 Left ventricular angiogram, AP (a) and lateral views (b). A jet of contrast is seen flowing through thickened aortic valve cusps. The ascending aorta is dilated. This is congenital valve stenosis in a neonate

THE ETIOLOGY OF CONGENITAL HEART DISEASE

The incidence of congenital heart disease in the general population is one in 100 live births. A small number (5%) are caused by a defect in the chromosomes of the infant who shows other evidence of this, for example, mongolism or Turner's syndrome. Possibly a further 3% are caused by single gene disorders which cause syndromes such as Marfan, Holt–Oram or Noonan.

Environmental causes can be clearly identified in only 2% of cases, when there is a clear association between exposure to rubella or drugs and the appearance of heart malformations. Drugs implicated with some certainty are thalidomide, hydantoin and lithium.

In over 90% of cases there is no clear cause and we assume that many factors are involved, including a small genetic predisposition acting together with one or more adverse environmental influences, such as drugs, virus infections and poor maternal nutrition. At present we cannot be sure that any drug is completely free from the possibility of causing congenital heart disease and no drugs should be prescribed during the first three months of pregnancy other than those which are absolutely essential for the mother's health.

ADVICE REGARDING FURTHER PREGNANCIES

The risks for further pregnancies in parents with one child affected by a congenital heart defect can be evaluated with some precision only when careful consideration is given to the specific features in their case. Thus, if there is congenital heart disease in near relatives then the possibility arises that there is a strong tendency to inheritance of heart disease. If either partner shows appearances of an inherited syndrome such as Noonan's syndrome or Marfan's syndrome then there is a high risk for further pregnancies. On the other hand, if there was a clear history of exposure to a known harmful drug, such as lithium (which carries a 10% chance of causing cardiac malformations and, in particular, Ebstein's anomaly of the tricuspid valve), or to rubella during the early stages of the pregnancy then the risk for further pregnancies should be low. This applies only if the harmful agent can be avoided in the future – the mother who requires to continue taking lithium for severe depression will have a high risk of having further children with congenital heart disease.

For the majority of parents who have one child with heart disease the risk of producing further affected children is less than 4% but there are obvious exceptions where the risk may be very much greater than this and some form of genetic counselling is advised before proceeding to a further pregnancy.

FURTHER READING

Nora, J. J. and Nora, A. H. (1978). *Circ.,* **57**, 205

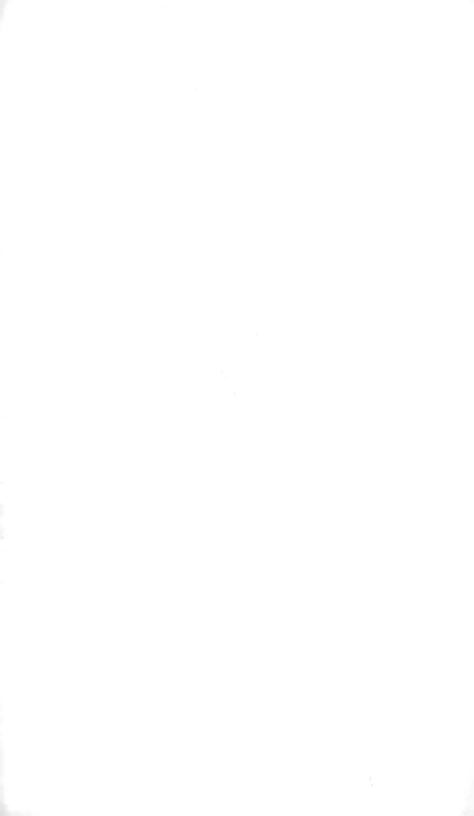

9
Long-term Problems

J. FLEMING and C. WARD

For some cardiac abnormalities effective therapy restores complete
normality and no regular medical supervision is required. Thus the
patient whose persistent ductus arteriosus has been ligated or whose
atrial septal defect has been closed may soon be discharged from
hospital outpatient attendance. There remains a large number of
conditions which modern management improves, but cannot be
said to have produced a complete cure, and regular follow-up is
essential. For many of these patients the use of sophisticated
diagnostic instruments is required to monitor progress, and regular
attandance at the cardiac outpatient clinic becomes necessary.

IMPLANTED CARDIAC PACEMAKERS

Many years of trouble-free normal life can be expected following
implantation of a modern lithium-powered pacemaker. The battery
is expected to last for at least eight years of continuous use but this
cannot be absolutely guaranteed and measurements of the battery
power are made every six months with the object of replacing the
pacemaker long before any clinically obvious failure of function
occurs. The exact time interval between successive pacemaker
impulses is measured electronically from the surface electrocardiogram, and the exact duration of the pacemaker stimulus measured
and noted. For one manufacturer's pacemaker typical figures are
850 msec and 0.5 msec respectively. These measurements are
obtained before and soon after implantation and any significant
deviation thereafter provides early warning of battery failure.

Wound breakdown

The pacemaker is usually implanted subcutaneously below the clavicle (Figure 9.1) or in the abdomen. It is always possible that the overlying skin will break down either because of trauma or low-grade infection, and the pacemaker then becomes visible. Such an event is uncommon but requires immediate admission to hospital for reimplantation of the pacemaker. The patient is in considerable danger at this stage because a serious infection can so readily spread from the tissues around the pacemaker to the heart and to the bloodstream. The site of implantation is checked routinely each time the patient visits the outpatient clinic and any signs of tenderness, inflammation or thinning of the skin should lead to immediate action to forestall a complete breakdown of the wound.

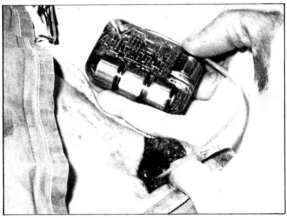

Figure 9.1 The incision over the cephalic vein with a pacemaker about to be inserted (courtesy of J.S. Wright)

Displacement of pacing wires

The wire leading from the pacemaker to the heart may become displaced, or break, or lose part of its surrounding insulation. These events, now fortunately uncommon, cause a complete failure of cardiac pacing and demand urgent admission to hospital where X-ray examination and analysis of the exact shape of the pacemaker impulse helps to identify the cause of the malfunction. So far, in

Britain there are very few examples of the 'pacemaker twiddlers syndrome'. First reported from the USA, this is a compulsive manipulation by the patient of his pacemaker which leads to a rotation and a winding up of the wire out of the heart.

Dizziness and syncope

Some patients report occasional attacks of dizziness or syncope yet no abnormality of function of the implanted pacemaker is detected at the pacemaker follow-up clinic. Possibilities include an intermittent failure of the cardiac pacemaker or episodes of tachycardia. The patient is fitted with a small tape recorder electrocardiograph which he carries strapped to his waist for 24 hours (Figure 9.2). The tape is then passed through a fast analyser and

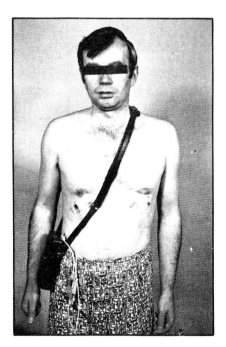

Figure 9.2 Patient equipped for continuous monitoring of the ECG (courtesy of J. S. Wright)

any abnormality of cardiac rhythm occurring during that 24 hours is identified.

Precautions

There is no restriction on air travel for the patient with an implanted pacemaker and little interference with his normal activities. He is warned to keep clear of high energy electrical fields such as radar and television transmission stations, and diathermy is usually best avoided during any surgical operations. Antibiotics cover for dental extraction, urethral catheterization and operations on the large bowel is highly desirable to minimize the risk of a blood-borne infection of the pacemaker.

CHRONIC RHEUMATIC HEART DISEASE

Mitral valve disease

Almost all patients with mitral valve stenosis will need long-term follow-up. Perhaps a young woman has been investigated and has been shown to have very mild mitral stenosis both on clinical grounds and following the results of chest X-ray, ECG and cardiac echogram. Despite her lack of symptoms she must be kept under review because the stenosis may well become more severe with the passage of time and there is always the possibility that a pregnancy will cause considerable problems. Apart from the special case of pregnancy there is little risk of sudden unexpected pulmonary edema or cardiac failure in the patient with known mitral stenosis. Using modern methods of assessment (Figure 9.3) we can measure the severity of the mitral stenosis with considerable accuracy and we can, therefore, arrange for all those patients with moderate to severe stenosis (Figure 9.4) to have cardiac surgery, either an 'open' mitral valvotomy or a mitral valve replacement – the type of operation is determined by the degree of degeneration and calcification in the diseased valve (Figure 9.5).

There remains a group of patients with significant, but not severe, obstruction at the mitral valve who are practically symptom

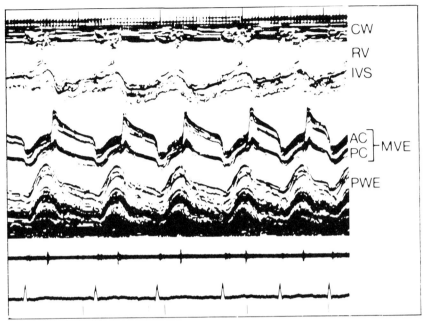

Figure 9.3 Echocardiogram of mitral stenosis. The various parts of the record are chest wall (CW), right ventricular cavity (RV), inter-ventricular septum (IVS), mitral valve (MVE), with its anterior cusp (AC), and posterior cusp (PC), and the posterior wall echo (PWE). The mitral valve is thickened, the posterior cusp moves anteriorly with the anterior cusp in diastole, i.e. paradoxically to the normal pattern (courtesy of A. McDonald)

free and in whom there is no danger of heart failure. In these patients who do not yet require cardiac surgery the one major danger is the possibility of systemic embolism. All these patients should be treated with long-term warfarin therapy and the dosage is controlled by regular checks of the prothrombin time. Provided that there are no strong contraindications to warfarin treatment this recommendation extends to include both the patients in atrial fibrillation and those in sinus rhythm. The latter can be expected to develop atrial fibrillation without warning and to be at greatest danger from systemic embolism during the first 48 hours thereafter.

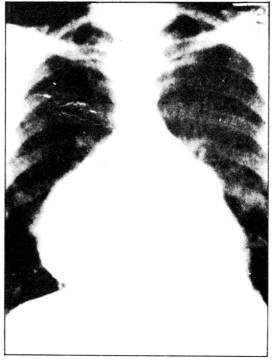

Figure 9.4   Chest radiograph showing the enormous heart of a man with severe, long-standing mitral valve disease. The left atrium alone is 60 per cent of the thoracic diameter and the right atrium was a small chamber perched on the anterior surface of the left atrium. This man never did really well after mitral valve replacement, dying one year later in intractable congestive heart failure (courtesy of J. L. Munro)

Aortic stenosis

For the adult patient with aortic stenosis the first essential is to determine the severity of the stenosis. Symptoms such as syncope or dizziness on exertion, chest pain or dyspnea would suggest that the valve is severely stenosed but it is not true to say that an absence of all symptoms indicates that the stenosis is mild. Sudden death can occur in a previously symptom-free patient. Clinical examination, including electrocardiography, chest X-ray and echo-cardiography, is supplemented by cardiac catheterization if there is any doubt regarding the severity of the stenosis. Severe aortic

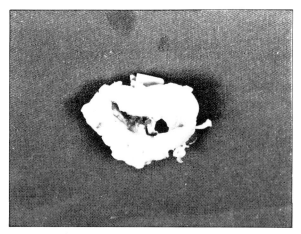

Figure 9.5 A severely stenotic and partially calcified mitral valve removed at operation. The grossly thickened and contracted cusps made it unsuitable for repair (courtesy of J. L. Munro)

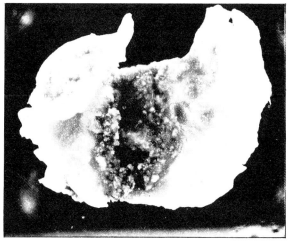

Figure 9.6 A heavily calcified and grossly stenosed aortic valve removed from a 41-year-old man. It was successfully replaced with an antibiotic sterilized homograft (courtesy of J. L. Munro)

stenosis (Figure 9.6) demands surgical relief either by aortic valvotomy or by aortic valve replacement and the surgical results are impressive. When the aortic valve stenosis is known to be of a mild degree then long-term follow-up at hospital is necessary, involving perhaps one or two visits each year. The electrocardiogram provides very valuable information in this condition, any sign of left ventricular hypertrophy developing, particularly if ST and T wave abnormalities appear, indicating that the valve stenosis has become severe.

Tricuspid valve disease

A diseased tricuspid valve presents a difficult problem in long-term management because surgical replacement of this valve does not usually give good relief from the chronic distressing symptoms of a high systemic venous pressure. The present practice, therefore, is to control the patient's symptoms for as long as possible by such measures as restriction of physical activities, control of ventricular rate with digoxin and reduction of venous pressure with diuretics and to refer for surgery only those patients with very bad tricuspid stenosis. We know that tricuspid valve disease can be difficult to diagnose when there is also significant disease of the mitral valve and the failure of some patients to do well following a successful operation on the mitral valve can often be attributed to hitherto unrecognized tricuspid valve disease.

CARDIOMYOPATHY

The patient with congestive cardiomyopathy usually presents in cardiac failure with a high venous pressure, swollen ankles, congested lungs and a large heart. The cause can be identified in only a small proportion of cases and occasionally, when the causative agent is removed, a complete recovery results. The cardiomyopathies caused by cobalt in beer or by sensitivity to drugs such as emetine can eventually return to normal. Some improvement can be expected where excessive prolonged consumption of alcohol is responsible and alcohol is given up completely. In others a hereditary cardiomyopathy occurs, linked with such conditions as Friedreich's ataxia and the Duchenne type of muscular dystrophy, or the cardiomyopathy is caused by amyloidosis, a collagen disease or some unidentified viral infection. All these tend to cause prolonged disability.

Initially it is important to establish that the cause of the heart failure is indeed a cardiomyopathy, i.e. a primary disease of a heart valve or systemic hypertension. Constrictive pericarditis must also be considered as a possible cause of congestive cardiac failure and all these conditions eliminated by as full investigation as necessary, perhaps including left ventricular angiography. Certainly, severe obstructive disease of the coronary arteries may present with the clinical picture of a cardiomyopathy and many causes hitherto considered to be caused by a primary cardiomyopathy have been shown on coronary arteriography to be the end result of coronary artery disease. The distinction between a cardiomyopathy and the congestive failure caused by coronary artery disease is not essential to the further management of the patient because coronary artery surgery has no place in treatment at this stage of the illness.

The initial response to treatment of a cardiomyopathy can be most gratifying but it should be remembered that for the majority of patients relapses into failure are to be expected. Management consists of severe restraint of physical activities, digitalization, oral diuretics to control fluid retention, with removal of any factors possibly adversely affecting the heart, such as toxic drugs and alcohol. The patient can usually return to work provided that this is sedentary in nature and further exacerbations of cardiac failure are treated by intensification of rest, perhaps with a week or two in hospital, and an increase in the diuretic therapy. Long-term anti-coagulants play a part in minimizing the incidence of pulmonary and systemic embolism but careful control is necessary in view of the changes in liver function caused by improvements and relapses in cardiac failure. Eventually the patient presents in chronic congestive failure with edema which is resistant to diuretics in very large dosage and at this stage some benefit may be obtained by lowering the peripheral vascular resistance, thus removing the pressure work of the heart. Oral hydralazine is perhaps the most useful drug in this respect but other hypotensive agents, including prazosin, have been used.

Hypertrophic obstructive cardiomyopathy

Hypertrophic obstructive cardiomyopathy is a particular form of inherited heart disease characterized by a selective hypertrophy of the interventricular septum. This hypertrophied septum obstructs the outflow of the left ventricle in mid-systole resulting in a small arterial pulse wave which is suddenly cut off. A characteristic feature of this condition is a small, sharp arterial pulse together with a systolic murmur, a gallop rhythm and considerable hypertrophy of the left ventricle. The diagnosis can be made clinically in the typical case and the echocardiograph is a most useful tool both in providing confirmation of the diagnosis in the florid case and in picking up patients with minor degrees of the abnormality. Sudden death, presumably caused by ventricular fibrillation, is not uncommon in patients with this disease and once the diagnosis has been established long-term management is essential. Present practice includes the long-term administration of a beta-blocking drug and the limitation of strenuous physical activities in an effort to prevent powerful contractive efforts of the left ventricle. Cardiac surgery offers an alternative approach to therapy: the cardiac surgeon divides the hypertrophied muscle and usually removes piecemeal parts of the hypertrophied septum. Left ventricular angiography will identify those patients who have localized areas of hypertrophy most suitable for surgical resection.

THE PATIENT AFTER SURGERY

Early convalescence can be interrupted by an illness with fever and chest pain, together with pleural and pericardial rub. This post-cardiotomy syndrome resolves with bed rest and analgesics, such as aspirin or indomethacin, with a few exceptions who require steroids to control a large pericardial effusion. Recurrences of this syndrome over a period of one year from the date of the operation are possible and are treated with a short period of bed rest.

Very many complications may occur, sometimes years after a successful cardiac operation, and usually the long-term follow-up of such patients is shared by the surgeon and the cardiologist.

Following heart valve replacement with a metal prosthesis the possible complications include embolism, hemolytic anemia and infective endocarditis. Long-term warfarin therapy is usually prescribed for these patients and in addition to routine prothrombin estimations the hemoglobin and blood film are studied at regular intervals. Antibiotics are given prior to procedures such as dental extraction and any sudden change in the patient's condition provokes an evaluation of the function of the valve: has it become infected, thrombosed or has it partly torn from its seating?

For women with prosthetic valves a successful pregnancy is possible with some increased risk both to the fetus and the mother. Heparin, which does not cross the placental barrier, is substituted for warfarin some weeks prior to delivery and, if the pregnancy is carefully planned, subcutaneous heparin may be used from the time of conception. For the pregnant woman there is a considerable advantage in having an xenograft valve, which does not require long-term anticoagulation, and this is the type of valve of choice for young women who require replacement surgery. The oral contraceptive pill, with its increased risk of thromboembolism, is best avoided completely when a metal prosthetic valve has been inserted.

After a successful coronary artery by-pass operation for angina treatment should continue for such factors as hypercholesterolemia, hypertension, obesity and diabetes. Any sudden reappearance of anginal symptoms may indicate the thrombosis of one or more grafts and the patient must then be considered for coronary angiography and possibly further surgery on his coronary arteries.

A complete cure by surgery of many congenital heart defects cannot be obtained and such patients are followed up regularly. Thus, resection of coarctation of the aorta lowers the blood pressure but over the years the pressure may rise and anti-hypertensive drugs are then required in some patients. Correction of Fallot's tetralogy may produce some pulmonary valve regurgitation and in many the ventricular septal defect is not completely closed. Such patients may eventually require further surgery. A few patients develop heart block years after surgery and then require an implanted cardiac pacemaker. This seems to be a problem particularly with an atrial septal defect of the ostium primum type.

10
Current Investigative Techniques

J. FLEMING and C. WARD

The cardiologist requires for his initial clinical assessment of the patient a straight anterior–posterior chest radiograph and a standard 12-lead electrocardiogram. These simple tests, together with a clinical history and clinical examination, provide the diagnosis and the basis for further management in the majority of patients referred to the cardiac outpatient clinic. Very detailed investigations of the heart can be undertaken if the diagnosis remains in doubt or in the course of preparation of a patient for cardiac surgery. This usually involves a thorough study of the precise anatomy and physiology of the heart lesion. The cardiologist attempts, by means of his preoperative investigations, to reduce to a minimum the incidence of surprise findings at cardiac surgery.

THE EXERCISE ELECTROCARDIOGRAM

Without any doubt, the exercise electrocardiogram can be a most useful investigation in the diagnosis and management of the patient with ischemic heart disease. Much effort has been involved in refining the test to increase both sensitivity and specificity, but no universally accepted method has yet emerged.

Most investigators agree that the electrocardiogram should be recorded continuously during exercise on a treadmill or on a bicycle ergometer (Figure 10.1) and that electrocardiographic monitoring should continue for at least five minutes after the end of exercise.

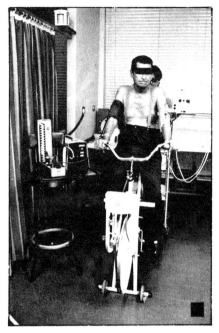

Figure 10.1 Exercise test performed on a bicycle ergometer with monitoring of the ECG and blood pressure (courtesy of M. N. Maisey and R. J. Wainwright)

Exercise is discontinued if chest pain develops, the blood pressure drops or the electrocardiogram shows marked ST segment depression. The appearance of a serious cardiac arrhythmia during exercise also indicates a positive exercise test. The usual practice is to attempt a submaximal exercise test by gradually increasing the severity of the exercise until the heart rate reaches 80% of the calculated maximum heart rate for the patient's age. Marked ST depression (Figure 10.2), e.g. more than 3 mm, strongly supports the diagnosis of ischemic heart disease. The problem of interpretation arises when one considers much smaller degrees of ST depression. If ST segment depression of 1 mm is considered a positive result then some normal patients will be wrongly diagnosed as having coronary artery disease. Furthermore, a negative exercise test performed under strictly controlled conditions does not exclude the presence of significant coronary arterial narrowing. Research

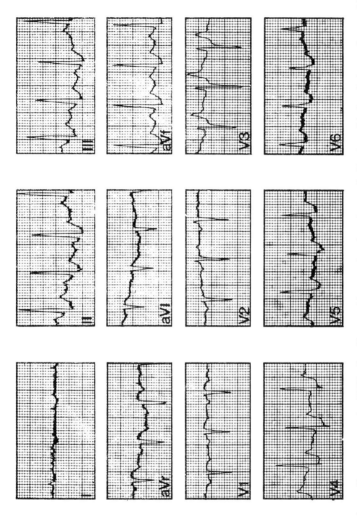

Figure 10.2 Immediate post-exercise ECG of a 40-year-old man, showing changes indicative of ischemic heart disease. Marked ST depression has developed in leads V_3 to V_6 (courtesy of A. J. Searle)

workers are attempting to increase the value of this test by recording from multiple chest leads during exercise and claim to have achieved an increase in sensitivity.

EXERCISE MYOCARDIAL SCINTIGRAPHY

This recently introduced test involves the injection of the radio-active substance thallium-201 into a peripheral vein during exercise. The patient is then positioned under a scintillation camera (Figure 10.3) and images from several views of the radioactivity of the heart muscle are obtained. Thallium-201 is not taken up by ischemic heart muscle and areas of myocardial ischemia are detected by the absence of radioactivity from the poorly perfused myocardium.

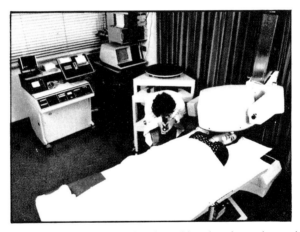

Figure 10.3   After exercise, the patient is positioned supine under a scintillation camera ready for cardiac imaging. Myocardial centering is checked with the persistence oscilloscope, which is seen on the upper left of the control (courtesy of M. N. Maisey and R. J. Wainwright)

Both the exercise electrocardiogram and the myocardial scinti-graphy test are non-invasive techniques for the diagnosis of coronary artery disease and are relatively safe provided that the exercise is strictly supervised in a cardiac laboratory with means of resuscitation, including a direct current defibrillator, immediately available. The exercise electrocardiogram is much less costly to perform than myocardial imaging but the latter is probably more sensitive and can provide information on the severity of coronary artery disease. It is claimed that a normal thallium-201 scintigram after maximal exercise excludes a stenosis of more than 50% in any major coronary artery.

CORONARY ARTERIOGRAPHY

All major cardiac centers now perform coronary arteriography and a precise knowledge of the anatomy of the coronary arteries together with the site of areas of stenosis or obstruction is, of course, essential before coronary artery surgery can be undertaken for the relief of angina. The investigation carries a small but by no means insignificant risk of death or serious complication, such as

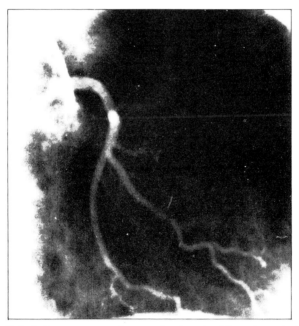

Figure 10.4 Left coronary angiogram showing the left main and circumflex arteries, but absence of left anterior descending artery, presumably totally obstructed at its origin (courtesy of D. G. Julian)

myocardial infarction and cerebral embolism. For this reason patients are very carefully selected and coronary arteriography is not usually performed merely to exclude the diagnosis of coronary artery disease. The patient with unexplained chest pain would normally be investigated fully by other means including exercise tests rather than subjecting him to coronary arteriography.

Coronary arteriography is performed via either the brachial or the femoral artery. A catheter is advanced under direct vision on the X-ray screen, into the ascending aorta. The operator then manipulates the tip of the catheter into the mouth of the left coronary artery, ensuring that he does not block the blood flow in the artery. Hand injections of 5 to 8 ml of radio-opaque contrast fluid are made and the passage of the fluid through the branches of the left coronary artery is photographed on high-speed cine (Figure 10.4). Multiple views are obtained by giving repeated hand injections with the patient in different positions relative to the X-ray cine camera. The catheter tip is then placed in the right coronary artery (Figure 10.5) and similar pictures obtained.

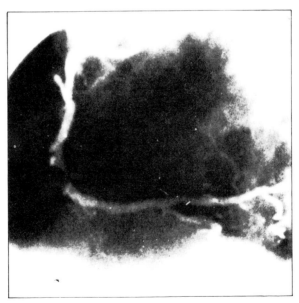

Figure 10.5 Coronary angiogram showing severely narrowed segment of right coronary artery (courtesy of D. G. Julian)

The examination almost always includes the taking of cine films after injecting about 40 ml of radio-opaque contrast medium through a catheter directly into the cavity of the left ventricle. From the left ventricular angiogram obtained, a good evaluation of left ventricular function can be made by watching the movements of the left ventricle. Localized areas of ischemia or infarction are seen to move little during ventricular systole. The ejection fraction of the left ventricle is calculated from the angiogram by estimating the left ventricular volume at end-systole and again at end-diastole. A good left ventricle has an ejection fraction of 0.7 or more and this means that the ventricle expels seven-tenths of its contents with each contraction.

The investigation of left ventricular angiography with coronary arteriography is performed under local anesthesia and requires hospital admission for at least 24 hours. The procedure takes less than one hour in the catheter room and is not particularly unpleasant for the patient. The mortality is well below 1% but some major complication can occur unexpectedly and this investigation cannot be regarded as perfectly safe even in the most experienced cardiac centers. Coronary arteriography is indicated when coronary artery surgery is under consideration for the relief of angina, and also as a preoperative investigation in patients requiring aortic or mitral valve replacement surgery. Some cardiologists recommend coronary arteriography in most patients who have angina or who have sustained a myocardial infarction because they believe that coronary artery surgery should always be advised for a severe stenosis of the left main stem of the coronary artery or where there are multiple lesions in the proximal parts of the coronary arteries. Quite apart from the huge work load that this policy would engender, there would be some morbidity and mortality in the large number of cases investigated. A preliminary screening procedure using exercise electrocardiography or myocardial scintigraphy is a reliable way of excluding left main stem stenosis and should be considered before proceeding to coronary arteriography.

ECHOCARDIOGRAPHY

The development of echocardiography for the examination of the heart has been one of the major advances in cardiology in the past 15 years. Short impulses of sound at a rate of 1,000 per second are directed towards the heart from a small microphone held against the skin of the chest wall. Echoes are reflected back to the microphone by almost all the heart structures, including the walls of the ventricles, the pericardium, the heart valves and the great vessels. The echocardiograph computes the time taken for the return of each echo and by this means estimates with precision the relative distances of each structure providing an echo from the microphone. The position of each structure is shown 1,000 times per second so that, in effect, a moving picture is obtained (Figure 10.6). The examination is completely painless and can be performed in 15 minutes. A great deal of valuable information is obtained from this examination but the moving picture produced is merely a representation of the movement of structures encountered by this very narrow, needle-like sound beam as it passes through the heart.

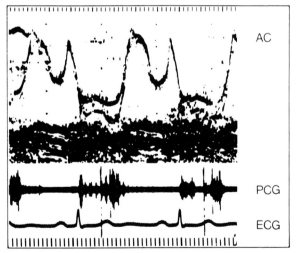

Figure 10.6   An example of mitral valve prolapse as revealed by echocardiography. The anterior cusp of the mitral valve (AC) opens in diastole, partially closes, and then flicks open again after the P wave of the ECG. The phonocardiogram (PCG) shows multiple systolic clicks and a late systolic murmur. In systole the posterior cusp (PC) separates from the anterior cusp (courtesy of A. McDonald)

The most recent development is the 'sector scanner' which incorporates a rapidly rotating head for the emission and collection of sound waves. Using this sector scanner, a moving cross-sectional picture of the heart is obtained which contains much more information than the original single beam echocardiogram.

The echocardiogram is readily recorded in the out-patient clinic and no preparation is necessary; except, perhaps, for infants in whom a mild hypnotic is helpful in minimizing patient movement. The patient lies supine or in the partial left lateral position and the operator holds the small head of the echo sounder against the skin of the chest wall in the third or fourth left intercostal space close to the sternum. In this area the sound waves can pass directly into the heart without encountering lung tissue. Good echoes cannot be obtained if there is lung tissue between the machine and the heart and this is one of the chief limitations of the technique. In patients with normal chests only a few areas are suitable for entry of the sound beam and in some cases of severe emphysema a satisfactory echocardiogram cannot be obtained at all.

The rapid movements of the anterior leaf of the mitral valve are first identified and a normal valve shows an amplitude of about 2.5 cm from the closed to the open position. Calcific mitral stenosis can be diagnosed when strong echoes are returned from the calcium in the mitral valve together with greatly decreased amplitude of movement. Mitral stenosis with normal valve mobility shows an anterior leaf with good mobility but with a slow rate of closure during diastole and the posterior leaf moves in the same direction as the anterior leaf throughout the cardiac cycle.

The operator next angles the beam downwards into the left ventricle and picks up echoes from the interventricular septum, the left ventricular cavity, the posterior wall of the left ventricle and the pericardium behind the left ventricle. The thickness of each of these structures can be measured, which provides a sensitive method of detecting asymmetrical hypertrophy of the septum, dilatation of the left ventricle or a pericardial effusion.

With the beam directed upwards the aortic and pulmonary valves can be studied and the left atrial cavity scanned for any echo from a left atrial myxoma. Further adjustment of the position of the transducer records the movement of the tricuspid valve.

When the sector scanner is used the patient experiences a slight vibration on his chest wall caused by the rapid rotation of the head of the machine. The two-dimensional cross-section provided by this instrument is particularly useful for detecting a ventricular septal defect, an atrial septal defect or for measuring the areas of the mitral and aortic valves when fully open. The severity of congenital defects can be precisely estimated.

CARDIAC CATHETERIZATION

Cardiac catheterization for measurement of pressures and oxygen saturations within the heart is often combined with angiography so that a detailed knowledge is obtained, both of the abnormalities in cardiac physiology and of the abnormal anatomy within the heart.

Catheterization of the right side of the heart is readily achieved via a vein in the arm or leg. Pressures and samples can be taken from the right atrium, the right ventricle and the pulmonary artery, and the catheter is then advanced until the tip wedges in any small branch of the pulmonary artery. The pressure recorded from this wedge position is very similar to the left atrial pressure and the finding of a very high wedge pressure in a patient with mitral stenosis could indicate that the stenosis is severe. Typical normal pressures and oxygen saturations obtained at catheterization are as follows:

Right atrium   2 mmHg
Right ventricle   25/2 mmHg
Pulmonary artery   25/10 mmHg
Pulmonary artery wedge   5 mmHg
Oxygen saturation 70% (mixed venous sample).

When an atrial septal defect is present the catheter can usually be passed across into the left atrium but, more importantly, a rise in oxygen saturation is detected in the right atrium caused by a flow of fully oxygenated left atrial blood through the defect into the right atrium. Similarly, a ventricular septal defect is detected by a rise in oxygen saturation at right ventricular level.

Left heart catheterization is accomplished by introducing the catheter through the femoral or brachial artery and manipulating the tip through the aortic valve into the left ventricle. Normal pressures are as follows: left ventricle – 120/0 mmHg; aorta – 120/80 mmHg. Aortic stenosis results in a raised left ventricular pressure as the left ventricle tries to overcome the resistance of the aortic valve and the pressure drop across the aortic valve provides a measurement of the severity of the stenosis. Left ventricular angiography can then be performed to show the narrowed aortic valve. Occasionally the obstruction to left ventricular outflow is below or above the aortic valve and this important information is clearly shown on left ventricular angiography. Left ventricular angiography will also reveal any regurgitation through the mitral valve and will provide information on left ventricular function.

ELECTROPHYSIOLOGICAL STUDIES

Most abnormalities of cardiac rhythm can be satisfactorily managed without the need for detailed electrophysiological studies.

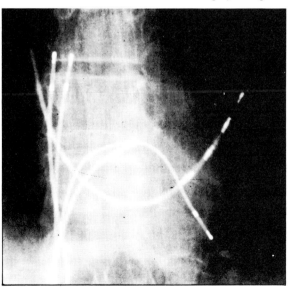

Figure 10.7 Radiograph showing the location of electrode catheters in the high right atrium, coronary sinus and right ventricle. The His bundle catheter is positioned against the septal leaflet of the tricuspid valve (courtesy of D. E. Ward and A. J. Camm)

A few patients, however, suffer repeated severe attacks of paroxysmal tachycardia which can be life-threatening and certainly disrupt the patient's normal work and every-day activities. In this type of patient control of the arrhythmia has usually been attempted without success by giving a variety of anti-arrhythmic drugs, such as quinidine, disopyramide, digoxin, propranolol and mexiletine, either singly or in various combinations.

These patients should be referred to an electrophysiologist who

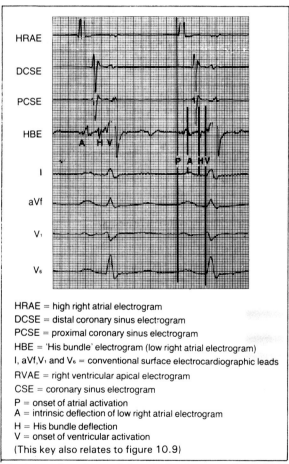

HRAE = high right atrial electrogram
DCSE = distal coronary sinus electrogram
PCSE = proximal coronary sinus electrogram
HBE = 'His bundle' electrogram (low right atrial electrogram)
I, aVf,V₁ and V₆ = conventional surface electrocardiographic leads
RVAE = right ventricular apical electrogram
CSE = coronary sinus electrogram
P = onset of atrial activation
A = intrinsic deflection of low right atrial electrogram
H = His bundle deflection
V = onset of ventricular activation
(This key also relates to figure 10.9)

Figure 10.8   A recording of normal sinus rhythm (courtesy of D. E. Ward and A. J. Camm)

will perform a very detailed analysis of the conduction system. This investigation requires hospital admission and the insertion of six or more electrode catheters into the heart from the peripheral veins (Figure 10.7). The electrical activity of the heart is then recorded simultaneously from the high right atrium, low right atrium, bundle of His, right ventricle and left ventricle (Figure 10.8). Single or multiple electrical impulses can be fired into the heart at various times in the cardiac cycle and the passage of these impulses analyzed from the multiple lead cardiac electrograms. During the examination, which may occupy several hours in the cardiac laboratory, the paroxysmal tachycardia can usually be initiated (Figure 10.9) and the response of the tachycardia to intravenous anti-arrhythmic drugs tested. The abnormality causing the

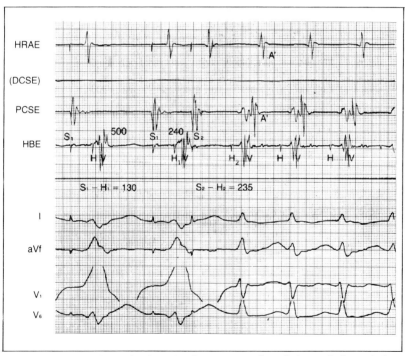

Figure 10.9 Regular pacing from the distal coronary sinus ($S_1 S_1$) results in marked ventricular pre-excitation. An atrial premature stimulus (S_1) blocks in the accessory pathway and conducts to the ventricles over the normal pathway with normal AV nodal delay. The impulse returns to the atrium (A) over the anomalous pathway and tachycardia is initiated. Courtesy of D. E. Ward and A. J. Camm

arrhythmia is diagnosed and the best drug for control is usually known by the end of the investigation. In some patients an accessory conducting pathway is found which responds poorly to drug therapy, or a damaged area of ventricular muscle is shown to be responsible for the arrhythmia. Cardiac surgery can be offered to these patients with the object of ablating the accessory conducting pathway or removing the damaged area of ventricular muscle. Recent experience has shown that very detailed electrophysiological studies are again required during surgery to ensure success in abolishing the arrhythmia.

THE USE OF CURRENT INVESTIGATIVE TECHNIQUES

Aortic valve stenosis

Echocardiography will show a poorly opening aortic valve with calcium in the valve if the patient is over the age of 40 years. Estimation of the severity of the stenosis is unreliable from the echocardiogram.

Left heart catheterization and coronary arteriography are usually necessary. Severe aortic stenosis is shown by a pressure difference of more than 40 mmHg between the left ventricle and the aorta at the peak of systole. Coronary angiography is performed in all patients requiring aortic valve replacement surgery because this is our only reliable method of detecting the presence of co-existent coronary artery disease. If severe coronary artery disease is revealed coronary artery by-pass grafting in addition to aortic valve replacement will be performed.

Aortic regurgitation

Echocardiography shows flutter of the mitral valve with normal movements of the posterior leaf and this is a reliable way of excluding a co-existent mitral stenosis. A rumbling mitral diastolic murmur is often heard in the presence of aortic regurgitation without there being any mitral stenosis, and the echocardiogram provides a simple way of showing the condition of the mitral valve.

Aortography shows the degree of aortic regurgitation and left ventricular angiography will exclude any mitral regurgitation. Coronary arteriography is performed if aortic valve replacement is under consideration.

Mitral stenosis

Right heart catheterization determines the severity of the stenosis from measurement of the wedge pressure and the pulmonary artery pressure.

Echocardiography gives information on the severity of the stenosis and the quality of the valve cusps.

Left ventricular angiography shows the condition of the left ventricle and also shows the presence and degree of mitral regurgitation.

Atrial septal defect

The echocardiogram shows enlargement of the right ventricular cavity and also shows an abnormal movement of the ventricular septum which is indirect evidence of an atrial septal defect. On the sector scanner a defect in the atrial septum is usually directly seen but false positive results are not uncommon.

Right heart catheterization shows the presence and degree of pulmonary hypertension and measures the size of the blood flow through the atrial septal defect. Angiography is difficult in this condition but may be helpful in showing anomalous pulmonary veins or in detecting an abnormal mitral valve in the less common ostium primum atrial septal defect.

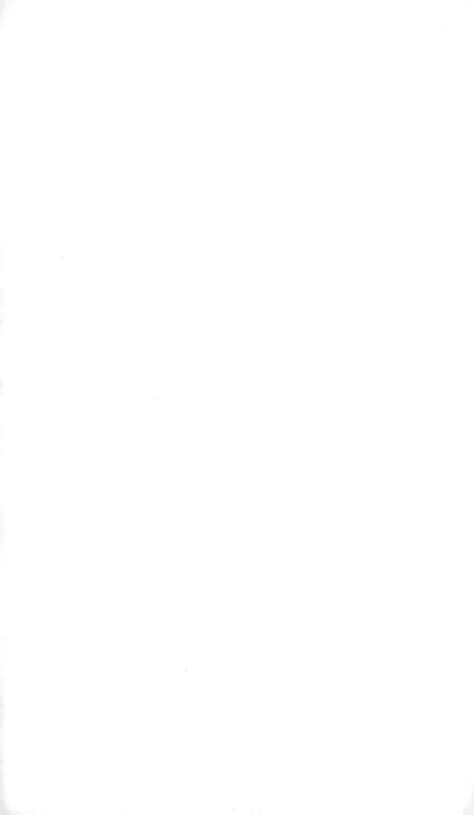

11
Managing Strokes

T. J. FOWLER

A stroke implies an area of brain damage caused by disturbance of the circulation and this damage is usually sufficient to destroy nerve cells. When, as a result, persistent signs remain a 'completed stroke' has taken place. Other terms also require explanation: 'stroke in evolution' or 'continuing stroke' indicate the slow development of neurological deficit, often in a step-wise fashion over a period varying from two to six hours (occasionally longer). Once the deficit has reached its peak a completed stroke has occurred.

Transient ischemic attacks (TIAs) are brief episodes of focal neurological disturbance with an abrupt onset and usually full recovery within several minutes. Most authors accept a duration of symptoms and signs of up to 24 hours, but if the signs persist beyond this a completed stroke is said to have occurred.

'Small strokes' imply short episodes of focal neurological upset which are of longer duration than a TIA and in which mild residual signs may persist. In many cases there is full recovery over a few days.

INCIDENCE OF STROKES

In Great Britain there are about 250 people per 100 000 population with new strokes each year. The mortality rate is 116 per 100 000 annually. About 80% of these strokes arise from thromboembolic cerebral infarction in which embolism from the heart plays an important role. Hemorrhagic lesions are responsible for the remaining 20%; 12% intracerebral hemorrhage and 8% subarachnoid hemorrhage (SAH). Of those who sustain an acute stroke, nearly one third die within a month and the survivors have an increased risk of further strokes.

A higher incidence of strokes occurs in the elderly and in this country nearly 75% of patients with acute strokes are admitted to hospital.

Survivors are often left with severe handicaps: about one half have significant motor deficits and only one third regain full independence. These figures emphasize the extent of the problem and the burden placed on medical resources.

PATHOLOGY

Traditionally the pathogenesis of strokes is divided into lesions caused by hemorrhage and those caused by occlusion of vessels through thrombus formation or embolism. Widespread atheroma in cerebral and extracranial arteries is often a contributing factor.

Hemorrhage

Hemorrhage occurs more commonly in hypertensive patients. Vessels may rupture with a massive catastrophic bleed, commonly producing a hematoma, or small microaneurysms, particularly in the basal ganglia and subcortical regions, may burst producing small areas of hemorrhagic softening, leading to microinfarcts or lacunes. These are also more common in hypertensive patients. Larger aneurysms may rupture with loss of blood into the subarachnoid space. This causes intense meningism with staining of the cerebrospinal fluid (CSF). Such bleeding may cause cerebral edema with marked arterial spasm and sometimes clinical deterioration.

Thromboembolic infarction

Thromboembolic infarction may arise from occlusion of arteries

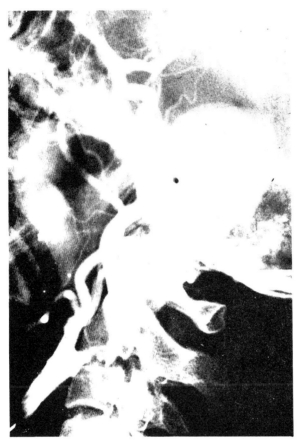

Figure 11.1 Lateral view of left carotid angiogram. The needle tip is in the common carotid artery and a tight irregular stenotic lesion can be seen in the internal carotid artery

often already diseased by atheroma. The arterial disease is usually widespread, but extracranial vessel occlusion has a relatively high incidence, particularly in normotensive patients. Emboli may arise from atheromatous ulcers and stenotic plaques, often in the carotid artery (Figure 11.1), and from the heart. In one series of 581 autopsies on patients with cerebral infarcts, 58% showed a possible source of emboli – 34% from the heart and 20% from the aorta and extracranial arteries (McCall 1975). In the heart, emboli may arise

Table 11.1 Precipitating causes of TIAs and strokes

1. Blood	Too 'thick'	Polycythemia
	Too 'thin'	Anemia
	Inflammatory	Arteritis, syphilis
	Chemistry	Diabetes, hyperlipidemia
2. Blood pressure	Too high	Hypertension
	Too low	Iatrogenic
3. Disorders of the heart		
a) Rate	Too fast	Supraventricular tachycardia
	Too slow	Heart block
b) Failure		Falling output
c) 'Ignition' upset		Varied rhythm
		'Sick sinus'
4. Embolic sources		
a) Cardiac		Infarcts, diseased valves
b) Extracranial arteries		Atheromatous ulcers
		Stenotic lesions
5. Mechanical compression		Vertebral arteries by
		osteophytes

from mural thrombus over a recent myocardial infarct or from valvular vegetations.

Many TIAs have a similar mechanism, with small fibrin–platelet emboli arising from atheromatous ulcers or stenotic lesions in extracranial vessels. They may also be secondary to falls in cerebral perfusion linked with disorders of cardiac rate or rhythm, to alterations in blood pressure, or to blood that is too thick (poly-cythemia) or too thin (severe anemia) (Table 11.1).

Inflammatory disease of arteries may rarely cause a secondary thrombotic endarteritis, e.g. in meningovascular syphilis or giant cell arteritis. There are also rare hemorrhagic disorders which may cause bleeding and the latter can follow the use of anticoagulant drugs.

DIAGNOSIS

The classical manifestations of a stroke in the territory of a carotid artery are striking, usually involving the sudden development of a focal neurological deficit, commonly a hemiparesis. This may be accompanied by hemisensory upset, an homonymous hemianopia or dysphasia, the last if the dominant hemisphere is involved. Varying patterns of deficit may reflect different branch occlusions or damage, but also reflect the efficacy of the collateral circulation from the circle of Willis. In the basilar territory, in addition to long tract involvement with a hemiparesis or hemisensory loss, there are commonly cerebellar features, often a Horner's syndrome and symptoms to suggest disturbance of the cranial nerve nuclei and their connections within the hindbrain.

The mode of onset of an acute stroke may give some help in diagnosis but clinicians' forecasts regarding pathogenesis are probably only correct in about 60% of instances, and they may also be incorrect in their anatomical placing of the site of damage.

Embolism has a very abrupt onset with neurological signs and often preserved consciousness. Hemorrhage, which may be precipitated by physical exertion or emotion, causes a rapid onset of signs, usually over the course of a few minutes. The signs are commonly accompanied by headache and vomiting and there is often early loss of consciousness. If blood enters the subarachnoid space meningism results, but about 15% of cases of hemorrhagic strokes have a clear CSF. A subarachnoid hemorrhage usually has a very sudden onset with severe headache, and is accompanied by florid meningism. Thrombotic infarction has a slower onset, usually over several hours, with a progressive deficit. This may be accompanied by a deteriorating level of consciousness, though about one third of patients developing a stroke may lose consciousness at or shortly after the onset. Some 4 to 10% of patients with strokes present with a fit. This is perhaps more common in those with hemorrhage.

Infarction may be accompanied by the development of cerebral edema which causes further deterioration, although this change may also reflect other causes, such as the development of broncho-pneumonia or even a mistaken initial diagnosis.

TIAs and small strokes are characterized by brief episodes of focal neurological deficit, their pattern being determined by the mechanism and territory involved. Occasionally small emboli can be visualized in the retinal vessels (Figure 11.2). Often there are no abnormal signs between attacks but examination may show

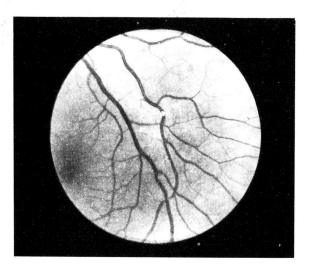

Figure 11.2   Retinal embolus seen as a small refractile body filling the lumen of the arterial branch

possible embolic sources in the heart or evidence of widespread arterial disease. A localized bruit in the neck over the carotid or vertebral arteries may indicate the presence of a stenotic lesion which is potentially treatable by surgery.

INVESTIGATIONS

It should be emphasized that 'strokes' are mistakenly diagnosed in some 3 to 5% of cerebral tumours and a number of other conditions should be considered, e.g. subdural hematomata, abscesses and infective processes, or metabolic disturbances. Investigations may be necessary for this reason but they may also help in directing attention to other features which may prevent further trouble or help to stabilize the cerebral circulation. Many factors determine the extent to which investigations are carried out, including the patient's age and physical state.

Table 11.2 indicates some of the useful tests which may help in management. A blood sample should be sent for a full blood count, ESR, urea, electrolytes and blood sugar. In younger patients a lipid profile and serological tests to exclude syphilis should be added. An ECG may reveal a possible cardiac source of emboli – ventricular

Table 11.2 Investigations for TIAs and strokes

1. Blood sample	Hemoglobin,
	PVC, white count
	ESR
	Urea and electrolytes, sugar
	Serum urate
	Lipid profile
	WR or equivalent
2. Measurement of blood pressure	
3. Cardiac assessment:	ECG, prolonged cardiac monitor[1]
4. Chest X-ray	
5. Skull X-ray	
6. Cervical spine X-ray[1]	
7. CSF examination[1]	
8. CT scan[1] (isotope if CT not available)	
9. EEG[1]	
10. Angiography[1]	

[1] If indicated

hypertrophy or susceptibility to a changing rate or rhythm. In some patients continuous ambulatory ECG monitoring may be necessary to detect paroxysmal arrhythmias. It should be remembered that after an acute stroke or subarachnoid hemorrhage a number of patients show ECG changes, usually T wave flattening or inversion and ST depression.

An EEG is a non-invasive test which may help to differentiate strokes from tumours. A persistent slow wave focus, particularly in serial recordings, favours the latter. After two to three weeks the EEG abnormality improves in most patients with a stroke.

Plain X-rays may be helpful in excluding other causes and a chest X-ray may show a primary tumour, metastases or cardiac enlargement. On skull films the pineal gland is calcified in nearly 50% of patients and shifts of this structure from the midline may indicate the presence of a mass lesion, sometimes a hematoma or even a tumour. If the pineal is not calcified ultrasound may be used to detect midline shifts.

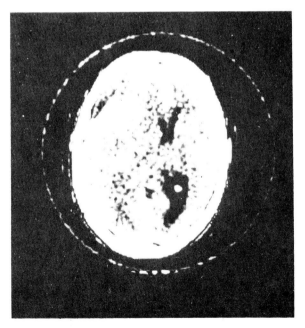

Figure 11.3 CT scan showing a left frontal subdural hematoma causing a shift of the ventricles to the right side

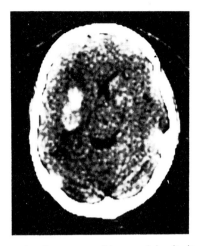

Figure 11.4   CT scan showing an area of increased density in the region of the left lentiform nucleus from an intracerebral hemorrhage

Computerized axial tomography (CT) scans have proved a major advance in the management of patients with strokes. Their use allows the exclusion of other conditions which may mimic a stroke, such as a subdural hematoma (Figure 11.3). They will show the presence of a hemorrhagic lesion (Figure 11.4) and indicate the rare hematoma which can be surgically evacuated. They are extremely helpful in the unconscious patient when the diagnosis is in doubt. The site of a bleed from a ruptured aneurysm may be shown (Figure 11.5) and the appropriate artery to be studied by angiography may be indicated. They will also show the presence of areas of cerebral infarction (Figure 11.6) and sometimes there may be evidence of more than one infarct which may not have been suspected clinically. In some patients there may be signs of widespread neurological damage often with an accompanying dementia. In some instances this damage may be due to multiple infarcts (Figure 11.7). Unfortunately, present resources do not allow all stroke patients to have access to CT scanning and largely for this reason isotope brain scans still prove valuable, particularly in the exclusion of metastases, benign tumours, such as meningiomata, and subdural hematomata.

The cerebrospinal fluid should be examined in patients with

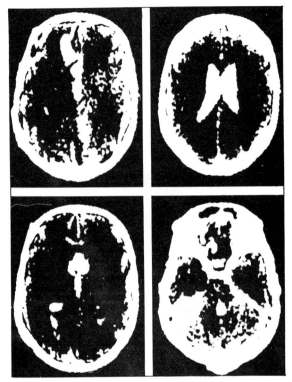

Figure 11.5   CT scan showing the rupture of a left anterior communicating artery aneurysm with hemorrhage into the left frontal region a), and into the lateral b), and the third c) and fourth d) ventricles.

meningism, particularly if infection needs to be excluded. The dangers of lumbar puncture in the presence of raised intracranial pressure should be remembered. Angiography is necessary to show the presence of aneurysms (Figure 11.8) or angiomata. It is also necessary to show atheromatous ulcers or stenoses (Figure 11.1) in patients with extracranial lesions where surgical disobliteration is considered as a means of stroke prevention. However, in those arteriopathic patients an increased morbidity results from this procedure. For this reason a number of non-invasive screening procedures based on Doppler ultrasound techniques are currently being evaluated.

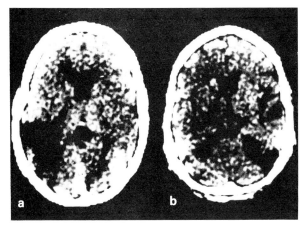

Figure 11.6   CT scans from two patients showing areas of cerebral infarction. In a) an area of low density can be seen in the left parietal region. In b) two smaller infarcts are shown: one in the right temporal region, the other in the right parietal region

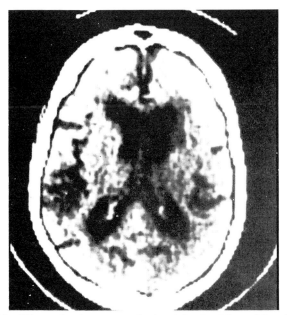

Figure 11.7   CT scan showing an area of reduced density at the periphery in the left temporal region and immediately adjacent to the side of the body of the right lateral ventricle. These are infarcts. The ventricles are widened and some large sulci are seen

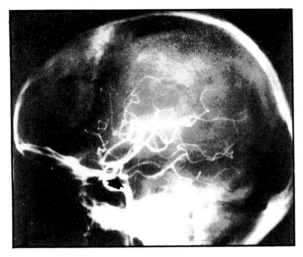

Figure 11.8   Lateral view of right carotid angiogram showing an irregular posterior communicating aneurysm (arrowed). The artery beyond this shows spasm. This patient had sustained a subarachnoid haemorrhage four days before this study

TREATMENT

Unfortunately, by the time doctors are called to most patients who have had a stroke, the damage is done. In a significant proportion there may be a depressed conscious level, diagnostic doubt, or inappropriate home conditions, so many patients are admitted to hospital.

Immediate resuscitative measures may be necessary depending on the patient's state and conscious level. In patients where deficits seem mild, early attention can be directed towards recognizing factors which may favour a recurrence or extension of damage with a view to their prevention.

In all patients it is worth writing down details of the initial assessment so that this is readily available for comparison in the face of changing level of consciousness or neurological signs. A number of signs are important, including the patient's best verbal and motor responses and the eyes – whether open and following or closed and unresponsive – the pupillary reactions and ocular movements. In addition, the pulse, blood pressure, respiratory rate and rhythm and temperature should be recorded. It is often necessary to follow these signs to assess improvement or deterioration. If the latter is occurring a number of possible causes require consideration. Is the diagnosis correct? Has cerebral edema developed or is there an expanding hematoma? Are secondary complications arising, such as bronchopneumonia or heart failure? Is there restlessness because of urinary retention? Recognition of such complications may allow their correction, but it should be emphasized that there is a small immediate mortality caused either by massive infarction or hemorrhage.

Acute measures

A depressed level of consciousness, or sometimes bulbar involvement, may cause acute airway obstruction which is potentially lethal. To overcome this the patient should be laid flat, semiprone and tilted slightly head downwards to allow any secretions to drain from the mouth. Suction may help to remove thick secretions or vomitus. Loose dentures should be removed and an airway may be inserted to help prevent the tongue from falling back.

Blood pressure and circulation

Some patients are hypertensive and this may have caused the stroke; in others there may be a reactive rise in blood pressure following the ictus. In elderly patients it is seldom necessary to lower the blood pressure, but in younger patients with a persisting high diastolic pressure and features to support previous sustained hypertension (retinal changes, cardiac enlargement on ECG or chest X-ray proteinuria) hypotensive therapy may be necessary.

Following an acute stroke vessels in a damaged area of brain seem to lose their usual vasomotor tone and this is probably why cerebral vasodilators have proved so disappointing.

In some patients, particularly the elderly, there may be coexistent heart failure. Treatment may help increase cardiac output and so improve cerebral perfusion.

After cerebral damage from infarction or hemorrhage,

secondary edema may appear. This may cause a deteriorating clinical state and can be difficult to differentiate from other causes, e.g. an expanding hematoma, although a CT scan may aid diagnosis. Various agents have been tried to reduce cerebral edema but all have certain drawbacks.

(1) *Diuretics* may reduce edema and cause a secondary diuresis; they may also lower blood pressure. Frusemide in a dose of 40 to 80 mg daily may be used.

(2) *Osmotic diuretics* include glycerol, which is rather unpalatable by mouth although it may be effective via a nasogastric tube or even an intravenous infusion. A few patients, however, develop hemolysis. Mannitol infused intravenously produces a rapid reduction in edema with a diuresis – unfortunately this is not sustained and rebound edema with clinical deterioration may follow.

(3) *Dexamethasone* is highly effective in reducing cerebral edema around metastases and tumours but seems less effective in cases of cerebral infarction. Conflicting reports have appeared and there are the usual risks of high dosage steroid treatment.

(4) *Low molecular weight dextrans* are thought to reduce plasma viscosity, blood sludging and platelet stickiness. One trial suggested that patients treated in this way had a lower mortality although many of the survivors had severe deficits (Matthews 1976).

The stroke patients who seem to be at greatest risk from edema are those in coma or with a depressed conscious level, a dense hemiplegia and failure of conjugate gaze towards the side of the limb weakness (indicating hemisphere damage extending into the frontal region – area 8); these patients may benefit from a diuretic and glycerol for 7 to 10 days (Oxbury 1975).

General care

Attention should be given to appropriate nutrition and hydration: oral feeding is usually feasible. In the elderly there may be problems with incontinence and constipation which require attention. Relatively immobile patients are more prone to develop secondary bronchopneumonia and pressure sores so that appropriate physiotherapy, posturing and turning are necessary. There is also an increased risk of deep vein thrombosis with secondary pulmonary embolism.

Acute cerebral hemorrhage

Patients suspected of having a subarachnoid hemorrhage should be admitted to hospital where the diagnosis can be confirmed by lumbar puncture. Angiography will be carried out in those in whom the clinical state (particularly the conscious level) is good and who are of appropriate age and fitness for surgery to be considered. If an aneurysm is found then the timing of surgery needs careful planning as the risks from rebleeding in the first few days need to be weighed against the increased surgical mortality and morbidity at that time. A CT scan may help to demonstrate the site of bleeding or the presence of a hematoma.

Epsilon aminocaproic acid (Epsikapron) or tranexamic acid (Cyklokapron) are inhibitors of the conversion of plasminogen to plasmin and so can prevent clot breakdown. Such clot may have formed in aneurysms that have bled and the use of these drugs may greatly reduce the incidence of rebleeding from ruptured aneurysms.

Where surgery is not feasible or no aneurysm is found, treatment by strict bed rest for five to six weeks is usual, followed by slow mobilization.

A sizeable intracerebral hematoma may follow a bleed in some patients. In certain circumstances this can be surgically removed with benefit. In patients in whom a primary intracerebral hemorrhage has occurred, early mobilization is possible. Often these patients are hypertensive and hopotensive treatment is necessary.

Rehabilitation

The major aspects of management in patients following a stroke are nursing them through the acute phase, mobilizing them early and encouraging them to regain their independence. The appropriate use of physiotherapy greatly helps the patient not only in balancing and starting to walk but also in using weak limbs where there may be accompanying sensory loss. Occupational therapy can help further and in those patients with persistent disability home visits to assess the best aids prove invaluable. In patients with dominant hemisphere damage speech therapy may also be helpful. Unfortunately a proportion of patients sustain damage with impairment of their higher mental functions and if this persists it may lead to continuing problems which result in the need for chronic care. About 20 to 30% of stroke survivors are permanently and severely disabled.

A proportion of patients who have sustained strokes may be nursed at home. These are often elderly patients or those whose deficit is mild and whose home conditions are good. The relatives may need help and instruction which can be augmented by visits from the practice nurse and home physiotherapy.

PATIENTS AT RISK: STROKE PREVENTION

It is in the recognition of the patient at risk that the general practitioner can exercise the greatest influence in stroke prevention. Patients who have sustained small strokes or who have had TIAs have a greater risk of developing subsequent strokes. Probably about 30% of patients who have had TIAs develop a completed stroke over the next five years: the incidence varies in different series. Carotid territory attacks carry a worse outlook. Certain precipitating causes are well recognized (Table 11.3) and, if identified, may be corrected. Atheromatous stenotic lesions or ulcers, usually near the origin of the internal carotid artery, are accessible to surgery and their removal may prevent strokes. Control of hypertension significantly reduces the incidence of strokes. Embolic sources within the heart may be treated with anticoagulants.

In some patients with a history of TIAs or small strokes the question of other types of prophylaxis has been raised. Their disease may be too widespread for or inaccessible to surgery. Anticoagulants may be of some benefit here particularly in the first six

Table 11.3   Risk factors in strokes

Hypertension
Cardiac disease
  a) failure
  b) ischemic heart disease
  c) embolic source   mural thrombus
                        valvular vegetations

TIAs
Previous strokes
Increased hematocrit
Lipid abnormalities (under age 55 years)
Diabetes mellitus
Smoking (males)
Oral contraceptive pill

months after a 'warning' episode. More recently it has been shown
in two trials that aspirin, which in a low dose reduces platelet
stickiness, may play a part in stroke prevention (Canadian Co-
operative Study Group 1978; Fields *et al.* 1977). These studies do
not provide a complete answer but the ease of treatment with few
side-effects make aspirin therapy attractive.

Abnormal blood lipids may play a role in premature development of atheroma. This has more significance in younger patients
(aged less than 55 years) where there is often a family history of
premature vascular disease.

Other risk factors include some which the patient can avoid, e.g.
smoking or the oral contraceptive pill. Recent attention has been
given to patients with an elevated hematocrit; lowering this
increases cerebral blood flow and may reduce the incidence of
strokes or ischemic symptoms.

These risk factors should also be considered in patients who have
sustained a completed stroke from which they have made a
reasonable recovery.

CONCLUSIONS

Particular attention should be paid to those at risk of developing
strokes; many such patients already have a history of premature
vascular disease. In those who have sustained a stroke, acute treatment should be commenced while investigations are carried out to

exclude other diagnoses. These investigations will also allow assessment of other contributory circulatory factors.

References

Canadian Co-operative Study Group (1978). *New Eng. J. Med.,* **299,** 53

Fields, W. S., Lemak, N. A., Frankowski, R. F. and Hardy, R. J. (1977). *Stroke,* **8,** 301

Matthews, W. B. (1976). In *Stroke,* 9th Pfizer Symposium (Edinburgh: Churchill Livingstone)

McCall, A. J. (1975). In Hutchinson, E. C. and Acheson, E. J. (eds.) *Strokes.* (London: W. B. Saunders)

Oxbury, J. M. (1975). *Br. Med. J.,* **4,** 450

Acknowledgement

The author is grateful to Mr J. Shilling for Figure 11.2, and to Dr C. Penney for prints of the CT scans. Figures 11.1 to 11.6 are taken from Fowler, T. J., *Strokes,* Update Postgraduate Centre Series, Update Publications, London, 1977.

12
Systemic Disorders and the Heart

C. WARD and J. FLEMING

The heart may be involved in a wide variety of conditions which are either generalized disorders or which primarily affect some other organ. The importance of these conditions is two-fold. First, cardiac involvement may be overlooked because the disease presents with features which direct attention elsewhere. Second, in other cases cardiac involvement may be dominant and the underlying pathology overlooked, as in some cases of thyrotoxicosis.

Many of the conditions which might be mentioned are rare. The aim here will be to discuss the systemic disorders associated with cardiac involvement which are most likely to be encountered by the family doctor. The subject can conveniently be considered in two sections. First, patients who present with one of the more common systemic disorders in which the heart may be affected, and second, the various ways in which heart disease may present without the underlying pathology being immediately obvious.

It should be remembered that atherosclerosis and hypertension are both generalized systemic disorders and that in a patient with, for example, a myocardial infarction, the disease may have affected other organs.

CONDITIONS WHICH CAUSE INCREASED CARDIAC WORK

Any disorder which calls for an increased cardiac output may bring to light previously occult heart disease or worsen a pre-existing condition. Anemia secondary to any cause can precipitate angina or cardiac failure, which may subsequently be 'cured' when the anemia is treated. Murmurs of valvular disease may be first heard whilst a patient is anemic and other ('hemic') systolic murmurs will disappear after adequate treatment. Severe infections, without directly involving the heart, have similar effects. Thyrotoxicosis, which in some respects comes under this heading, will be considered below.

CONGENITAL HEART DISEASE

Many chromosome disorders have widespread effects. Most of those which involve the heart are rare. However, Down's syndrome (Mongolism) affects one in 600 to 700 live births and is much more common with increasing maternal age. Congenital heart disease occurs in about 40% of these cases. Defects of the atrial or ventricular septa, alone or in combination, account for 75% of lesions. Patent ductus arteriosus is next most frequent. Turner's syndrome (Figure 12.1) is a much less common chromosome defect but the patient can be readily recognized. All are women and have webbing of the neck, hypertelorism and amenorrhea. Almost three-quarters of these patients have coarctation of the aorta.

The rubella syndrome causes widespread damage and many affected patients die in infancy. Approximately one third of those who survive have congenital heart disease. This usually takes the form of pulmonary stenosis, but patent ductus arteriosus, ventricular or atrial septal defect and Fallot's tetralogy have all been observed.

THYROID DISORDERS

Thyrotoxicosis

The increased metabolic rate which results from thyrotoxicosis can place an excessive burden on the heart especially in the elderly. Thyrotoxicosis may cause the following, singly or in combination:

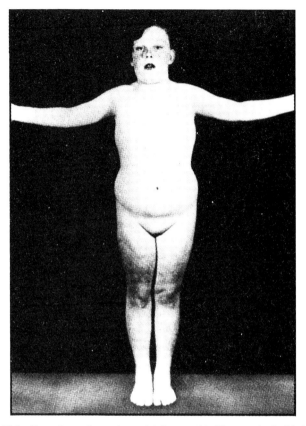

Figure 12.1 Turner's syndrome (gonadal dysgenesis). Note stocky build, laterally placed nipples and increased carrying angles at the elbows

(1) Atrial fibrillation.
(2) Cardiac failure.
(3) Angina.

Each of these effects may be difficult or impossible to control until the underlying thyroid disorder is corrected. Thus recognition of the cause is essential for adequate treatment. In most cases the clinical diagnosis of thyrotoxicosis is obvious: the symptoms and signs include a warm dry skin, tremor, prominent eyes, thyroid enlargement and a bruit, weight loss (often despite an increased

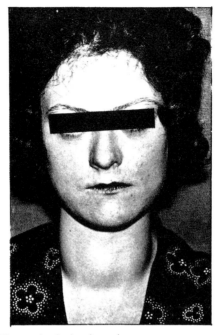

Figure 12.2   Thyrotoxicosis showing goitre

appetite) and irritability (Figure 12.2). Patients who are not in
atrial fibrillation have sinus tachycardia and a full bounding pulse.

Atrial fibrillation (Figure 12.3) is more common after the age of
45 years, especially when there is a pre-existing heart disease. The
ventricular rate may be very rapid. However, up to 50% of patients
revert to sinus rhythm when the thyrotoxicosis is suppressed.

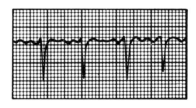

Figure 12.3   Atrial fibrillation. The base line shows fast irregular undulation from
the fibrillating atria. The ventricular rate is fast and irregular

Cardiac failure is not simply a reflection of the rapid heart rate or of pre-existing heart disease. It is apparent that in between one third and one half of all patients there is direct heart muscle damage, i.e. a cardiomyopathy (see below). Because of the nature of the disorder, patients with thyrotoxicosis and heart failure have a paradoxically hyperdynamic circulation. This is reflected in the full pulse, warm extremities and normal or near-normal jugular venous pressure. These features in a patient with heart failure should always lead to suspicion of hyperthyroidism.

Diagnosis and treatment

Assay of serum T4 in conjunction with a T3 uptake test and free thyroxine index will usually demonstrate the diagnosis. Treatment may take three forms, as follows:

(1) Antithyroid drugs.
(2) Radioactive iodine.
(3) Surgery.

The method of treatment chosen depends largely on the age of the patient and on the size and nature of the thyroid gland. Until therapy takes effect the patient should have symptomatic treatment, e.g. for cardiac failure. The beta-blocker drugs are valuable for helping to control the heart rate and for suppressing the peripheral effects of excessive sympathetic activity.

Myxedema

The metabolic rate is low in myxedema and consequently the cardiac output is reduced. However, whether or not myxedema causes cardiac failure is debatable since it is likely that the reduced output is sufficient for the decreased demands. On the other hand, hypothyroidism predisposes to atherosclerosis and replacement therapy quite often precipitates angina. Thus the significance of the heart in myxedema is related more to the effects of treatment than to the disease itself.

The features of myxedema are legion but develop insidiously and may easily be overlooked. They include aches and pains,

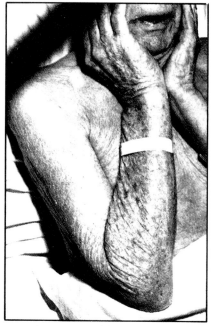

Figure 12.4 Dryness and coarseness of the skin in myxedema

menorrhagia, dry skin (Figure 12.4), loss of hair, weight gain, constipation, mental changes, edema and anemia (Figure 12.5). There is often a bradycardia, although some patients have atrial fibrillation. The chest radiograph usually shows cardiomegaly. In the majority of cases this is due to a pericardial effusion and not to cardiac failure.

Diagnosis and treatment

Serum T4 and the T3 uptake test (as in hyperthyroidism) will usually indicate whether or not the clinical diagnosis is correct. In doubtful cases the serum TSH concentration will almost invariably be raised if myxedema is present.

Treatment consists of replacement therapy using L-thyroxine 100 to 200 microgrammes/day (Figure 12.6). In patients with pre-existing heart disease and in the elderly much smaller doses may be

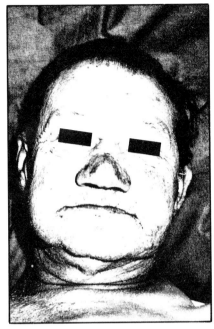

Figure 12.5 The typical facial appearance of myxedema with puffiness especially around the eyes. This is due to deposition of a mucoid substance

Before T$_4$

2 months after T$_4$ 0·1 mg/day

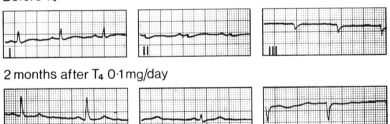

Figure 12.6 The ECG may be abnormal in hypothyroidism, but the changes are usually nonspecific. There is some flattening of the T-waves and decreased amplitude. These changes are reversed after treatment with thyroxine (T$_4$)

needed initially to avoid the precipitation of angina, heart failure or myocardial infarction. The addition of standard treatment for failure and angina is indicated when these complications occur.

Even with these precautions, correction of myxedema may have to be carried out with great caution.

INFECTIONS

Bacterial

At one time purulent pericarditis and 'septic myocarditis' were common complications of septicemia but since the introduction of antibiotics they are rare. Occasionally cases caused by staphylococci are still seen and have a poor prognosis. Far more important is the occurrence of infective endocarditis (subacute bacterial endocarditis) which may follow even apparently trivial infections in patients with underlying valve disease. Previously patients with known rheumatic heart disease were the usual victims but nowadays more and more cases occur in older patients without documented valve disease. Any patient with a heart murmur and evidence of systemic infection should be regarded as having infective endocarditis until proved otherwise. The mortality is still 30% and the best way to improve the prognosis is to hospitalize the patient without delay so that appropriate antibiotics, based on *in vitro* testing of organisms grown from blood cultures, can be given before irreversible valve damage occurs.

Viral

Nowadays viruses are the commonest group of organisms which infect the heart. The Coxsackie group B viruses are most frequently involved but almost all the viruses which infect man have been implicated at different times. Viral heart disease takes the form of myocarditis, pericarditis or, as is usual, a combination of the two – hence the term myopericarditis. The patient may, therefore, present with pericardial pain, cardiac failure or an arrhythmia. Clinical findings in the heart give no clue to the etiology but other symptoms and signs may do so. There is often a history of an upper respiratory tract infection or of an influenza-like illness during the preceding seven to 10 days and on examination there may be a rash or lymphadenopathy. Two blood samples taken seven to 10 days apart should be sent to the virus laboratory for testing, and a throat swab and stool specimen should be sent for culture with the first blood sample. However, the causative organism is often not found and the diagnosis must be based on clinical grounds.

Treatment is symptomatic but those who are clearly ill should be admitted to hospital for observation. Full recovery is usual but this may take several months. Occasionally a patient dies from intractable cardiac failure or from an arrhythmia: others develop chronic cardiac failure and remain disabled. Patients who have had pericarditis may have one or more recurrences.

NUTRITIONAL AND DRUG-INDUCED DISORDERS

Illness due to malnutrition is not uncommon in the US especially amongst the elderly living alone. A form of beriberi caused by deficiency of the group B vitamin, thiamine, is the best known disorder in this group which affects the heart. The usual consequence is high output cardiac failure which results from a reversible disorder of carbohydrate metabolism. Thus, as in anemia and thyrotoxicosis, the patient may present with a bounding pulse, warm extremities and peripheral edema. The findings are often incorrectly attributed to coronary artery disease. This is regrettable since treatment with thiamine is simple and dramatically effective.

Thiamine deficiency is a major cause of heart disease in alcoholics. However, excessive alcohol intake also damages the heart: in many cases both factors operate. Alcoholic cardiomyopathy classically occurs in middle-aged men who drink to excess for many years. Many are not typically alcoholic in that their drinking does not interfere with their work or family life and they may only rarely get drunk. Early complaints are breathlessness and palpitations. Atrial fibrillation is common but sinus tachycardia associated with ventricular ectopic beats is said to be particularly suggestive. Cardiac failure eventually occurs and, unless alcohol is withdrawn, becomes intractable.

A number of systemically administered drugs, in addition to those used primarily to treat cardiac disorders, may adversely affect the heart. Drugs which cause arrhythmias – notably sympathometic amines and tricyclic antidepressants – have been

discussed in Chapter 6. These same drugs occasionally cause myocardial damage. The ability of some drugs to cause hypertension
should not be forgotten. The best known example of this is the
hypertensive effect of taking a monoamine oxidase inhibitor antidepressant in combination with tyramine-containing foods, such as
cheese. A tricyclic antidepressant should not be given to a patient
taking a sympathomimetic drug since this combination may also
cause hypertension. In general terms, the antidepressant drugs
should be avoided in patients with known heart disease.

RHEUMATIC AND COLLAGEN DISORDERS

In some respects, acute rheumatic fever may be regarded as a
rheumatic disorder. However, unlike the chronic conditions we will
consider it would, were it not for the effects on the heart, be a
relatively trivial self-limiting illness.

Rheumatoid arthritis is common and the longer the disease is
present, the greater are the chances of cardiac involvement. Myocardial, pericardial and valvular disease have all been described –
up to 50% of patients have some cardiac complication. The heart
may also be affected in ankylosing spondylitis: aortic regurgitation
is the best known complication.

Systemic lupus erythematosus and periarteritis nodosa are the
best known of the collagen disorders: they are not common and
merit only brief mention here. The commonest cardiovascular
effect of both conditions is hypertension. In systemic lupus
erythematosus, pericarditis is common. Valve lesions also occur
frequently but very rarely cause problems.

Marfan's syndrome is an inherited disorder of connective tissue
characterized by long limbs, depressed sternum, kyphoscoliosis and
dislocated lenses. Complications include aortic regurgitation and
dissecting aortic aneurysms.

NEUROMUSCULAR DISORDERS

There are several forms of muscular dystrophy. The commonest
form affects boys only and usually proves fatal within a few years.

The heart is affected in up to 90% of patients. Sinus tachycardia is common but symptoms of cardiac failure are unusual. This contrasts with Friedreich's ataxia, the other hereditary neuromuscular disorder commonly associated with heart disease. In this condition death from cardiac failure frequently occurs within 20 years of the onset of neurological symptoms.

Perhaps the most important point to remember with respect to the rheumatic and neuromuscular disorders is that it should not be automatically assumed that a patient's breathlessness is due to the strain imposed by diseased joints or weakened muscles: the patient should always be examined for evidence of heart disease.

PERICARDITIS AS A PRESENTING SYMPTOM IN SYSTEMIC DISEASE

Inflammation of the pericardium usually presents with pericardial pain. This pain characteristically has two elements to it as follows:

(1) A more or less continuous restrosternal pain.
(2) Exacerbation of the pain by coughing, deep breathing and changes in posture.

The pain may persist for several days. On examination, the hallmark of pericarditis is a superficial scratchy sound (pericardial rub) which may be heard in systole, diastole or both. It is sometimes erroneously diagnosed as a heart murmur.

Pericarditis tends to be equated with a viral etiology but there are several other causes numerically more important, such as the collagen disorders, which must be kept in mind. In one large review (Griffith and Wallace 1953), viral infections accounted for 10 to 15% of cases as did rheumatic fever, septicemia, myocardial infarction and uremia. Malignant disease was responsible for about 10%. In these latter cases the primary tumor may be difficult to find. The commonest sites are lung and breast followed by the lymphomas. Malignant pericarditis is often associated with hemo-pericardism and intractable arrhythmias.

Reference

Griffith, G. C. and Wallace, L. (1953). *Dis. Chest,* **23**, 282

13
Current Therapy

GEOFFREY MAIDMENT and IAN JAMES

This chapter covers four main areas of therapy for cardiovascular disease: angina, hypertension, heart failure and arrhythmias. Emphasis has been placed on those aspects of therapy which the GP is likely to initiate.

MANAGEMENT OF STABLE ANGINA

Angina is one of the commonest features of ischemic heart disease. Chronic angina with predictable precipitating factors (stable angina) is usually managed by the general practitioner. Efforts must be made to keep the patient pain-free by optimal use of drugs but coronary artery surgery is considered if angina remains a serious problem.

Remediable factors

Attention should be paid to risk or aggravating factors as well as to treatment of the pain itself. Hypertension should be treated with a beta-blocker as the first line agent. The diagnosis of 'angina' provides a powerful incentive for the patient to stop smoking and weight loss must be encouraged in the obese.

Underlying cardiac disease may produce angina. Aortic stenosis accounts for only a small percentage of cases of angina but is surgically remediable. Other conditions, such as cardiomyopathy, anemia and thyrotoxicosis, may cause or aggravate angina.

General measures

Physical exercise to a point short of precipitating pain should be encouraged. However, activities which are regularly found to provoke pain, despite adequate drug therapy, should be avoided. This may mean that the patient must modify his lifestyle by walking more slowly and avoiding heavy meals. Cold weather may precipitate angina but wrapping up in warm clothes may prevent it.

The patient may need to change his occupation if his work is unsuitable (e.g. manual laborer) but hasty decision may be regretted, particularly as a substantial proportion of patients become free of angina (up to 30% at six months). Drivers of heavy goods and passenger service vehicles and airline pilots are obliged to inform the licensing authorities and must change jobs.

Avoidance of competitive activity and sudden bursts of effort, such as heavy lifting or pushing a car, is advisable. Anxiety may aggravate symptoms and should be managed by reassurance and beta-blockade.

TREATMENT OF THE ACUTE ATTACK OF ANGINA

(1) *Stop activity.* The patient should be advised to stand still or sit down as soon as discomfort starts. 'Walking through' the pain should be discouraged as it may lead to ventricular arrhythmia or myocardial infarction.

(2) *Glyceryl trinitrate.* This may be the only drug required in mild cases. Its main action is probably on peripheral vessels causing lowered peripheral resistance, venous return and blood pressure; thus heart work is reduced.

The drug should be taken sublingually as it is ineffective when swallowed. Its onset of action is rapid and most patients are relieved of pain within five minutes. The drug's effect persists for up to 45 minutes.

The patient should be instructed to carry the tablets with him and to suck a tablet when he feels pain coming on. When first starting on the tablets it is advisable that the patient is sitting or reclining as syncope occasionally ocurs from a drop in blood pressure. After relief has been obtained the remainder of the tablet can be swallowed or discarded. Chewing a tablet and allowing small pieces to dissolve in the saliva may produce more rapid pain relief. To obtain maximum benefit a tablet should be sucked just prior to activities which the patient knows by experience are likely to precipitate angina.

The patient should be warned about the headache which often accompanies the use of glyceryl trinitrate. It should be explained that this is harmless and often lessens with continued use. If this symptom is a problem it may be reduced by substituting a smaller dose (e.g. 0.3 mg) for the standard (0.5 mg) or discarding the tablet as soon as the chest pain lessens. Patients should be reassured that they can take as many tablets a day as they need.

Prevention of attacks

Beta-adrenoceptor blocking drugs

Beta-blockers have revolutionized the management of angina and should be tried in all patients having regular attacks of pain. They reduce the oxygen requirement of the heart by reducing heart rate and velocity of contraction as a direct result of beta-blockade.

Propranolol continues to be the most widely used drug. It should be taken three or four times a day for optimum effect in angina. It is recommended that therapy should start with a small dose (e.g. 10 mg t.d.s.) and build up dosage gradually. Lack of therapeutic response may indicate inadequate dosage. The dosage should be tailored to the individual patient and be increased until optimal control of symptoms is obtained, usually between 20 mg and 160 mg thrice daily. Most treatment 'failures' are due to inadequate dosage or misdiagnosis.

Production of sustained release preparations (see Table 13.1) and long-acting drugs, such as atenolol, have made feasible once-daily medication.

Unwanted effects. Caution should be exercised in those patients with uncontrolled heart failure, obstructive airways disease, peripheral vascular disease and conduction defects, which can be

Table 13.1 Beta-blockers for use in the management of angina and hypertension

Drug	Proprietary name	Cardioselective	Recommended dosage regime	
			Angina	Hypertension
Acebutolol	Secretal	±	100 to 400 mg twice daily	200 to 800 mg once daily
Atenolol	Tenormin	+	100 mg daily	100 mg daily
Metoprolol	Betaloc, Lopressor	+	50 to 100 mg twice or thrice daily	100 to 400 mg once daily
Oxprenolol	Trasicor	–	40 to 160 mg thrice daily	80 to 320 mg once daily
Oxprenolol (slow release)	Slow Trasicor	–	160 to 480 mg once daily	160 to 480 mg once daily
Propranolol	Inderal	–	40 to 160 mg thrice daily	80 to 240 mg twice daily
Propranolol (slow release)	Inderal-LA	–	160 to 320 mg once daily	160 to 320 mg once daily
Sotalol	Betacardone, Sotacor	–	160 to 480 mg once daily	160 to 480 mg once daily
[1]Metoprolol + hydrochlorothiazide	Co-betaloc	+	—	1 to 1½ tablets twice daily
[1]Oxprenolol (slow release) + cyclopenthiazide	Trasidrex	–	—	1 to 3 tablets once daily

[1] N.B. Combined preparation with a thiazide

aggravated by beta-blockade. Cardioselective drugs (such as metoprolol or atenolol) may provoke less bronchospasm in asthmatics and less impairment of the response to hypoglycemia and insulin-dependent diabetes.

The risk of heart failure has probably been over-emphasized but beta-blockers should be used with care in patients with cardiomegaly, a gallop rhythm or history of heart failure. Pretreatment with diuretics and digoxin may prevent this complication. Less serious unwanted effects, such as lethargy, nightmares, and gastrointestinal disturbances are usually tolerable. Abrupt withdrawal of beta-blockers must be avoided as there are reported instances of worsening angina and myocardial infarction. There is little to choose between the drugs in their therapeutic effect but if one does not suit it is worth trying another.

Long-acting nitrates

Recent carefully conducted studies have shown clear benefit of these compounds in angina. They are often used with a beta-blocker and their effects are additive.

(1) *Isosorbide dinitrate (Isordil).* When swallowed, the effect of isosorbide dinitrate is evident after about 30 minutes and lasts for about five hours. Larger doses are now used than in the past, usually between 40 and 120 mg daily in four divided doses. It may be taken sublingually, when its effects are evident in five minutes and last for about one hour.

(2) *Sustained release trinitrate (Sustac, Nitrocontin).* Recent work has shown the efficacy of these preparations. The duration of action is about 4 hours and the recommended dosage is 2.6 to 12.8 mg three times daily.

Other drugs

Nifedipine (Adalat). This is a newer antianginal agent which probably acts by protecting the heart against excessive oxygen utilization during physical activity. It is a potent calcium antagonist. The drug also causes peripheral vasodilatation and thus reduces peripheral resistance and heart workload.

The usual dose is 10 to 20 mg six-hourly. For relief of pain, the capsule may be bitten and the contents held in the mouth but it is slower in action than glyceryl trinitrate. It may be used with beta-blockers or nitrates. Unwanted effects similar to those of the nitrates occur, such as headache and dizziness, but it is generally well tolerated.

Perhexilene maleate (Pexid) is also effective in angina but reports of peripheral neuropathy have diminished enthusiasm for this drug.

Miscellaneous. Verapamil (Cordilox) and prenylamine (Synadrin) are occasionally useful but have not gained widespread acceptance. Anticoagulants, dipyridamole (Persantin) and clofibrate (Atromid) are no longer recommended in the management of angina.

Coronary artery surgery

In a high percentage of patients angina can be relieved by coronary bypass surgery and quality of life is often dramatically improved. Selection of patients can be difficult but severe angina in younger patients responding poorly to medical therapy is a clear indication, providing that the coronary anatomy is suitable and left ventricular function adequate.

The effect on prognosis is unclear, although in patients with severe left main coronary artery disease survival rates are improved. The risks of angiography and surgery are low but must be weighed against potential benefits.

UNSTABLE ANGINA

Angina which rapidly increases in severity or frequency may indicate impending myocardial infarction and is best treated in hospital. Bed rest, sedation, beta-blockade and nitrates are appropriate therapy.

MANAGEMENT OF HYPERTENSION

Most patients with raised blood pressure have 'essential' or primary hypertension. Hypertension due to specific underlying causes is more rare and will not be discussed here.

MANAGEMENT OF PRIMARY (ESSENTIAL) HYPERTENSION

The care of hypertension is a joint exercise between doctor and patient. To ensure co-operation there must be thorough discussion of the nature of treatment at the outset. A simple regime with few side-effects encourages compliance. Such a regime is shown in Figure 13.1.

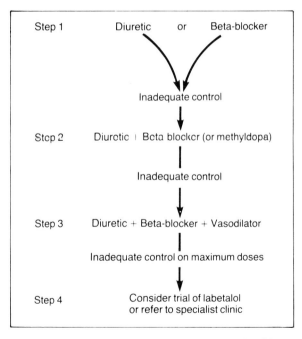

Figure 13.1 Suitable regime for routine management of mild to moderate hypertension

General measures

General measures, such as stopping smoking, weight reduction, treatment of diabetes and of hyperlipidemias, must not be forgotten. Severe salt restriction is not generally recommended but a high salt diet should be avoided particularly in more severe cases. Drugs known to cause raised blood pressure, such as oral contraceptives, steroids and phenylbutazone should be avoided.

Drugs for control of blood pressure (see Tables 13.1 and 13.2)

Diuretics

Thiazides. These are the drugs of initial choice as they are well tolerated and may alone control hypertension. The mechanism of action is uncertain but they produce a salt and water diuresis and reduce peripheral resistance.

Although usually considered 'mild' antihypertensives they are worth trying alone first, even when blood pressure is considerably raised, as some patients show a substantial response. There is little to choose between the many thiazides available – bendrofluazide is well tried and cheap.

Nothing will be gained from giving thiazides more frequently than once daily or in higher doses. They have a long duration of action and should be taken in the morning to avoid nocturia.

Unwanted effects include increased potassium loss from the kidneys but on an adequate diet no potassium supplements should be required. However, in the elderly, those with cardiac or renal disease and those on digoxin or steroids, potassium supplements may be important. It is advisable to check plasma potassium after about three months of therapy and again after a year.

Hyperuricemia occurs and gout may be precipitated. Allopurinol in combination with a thiazide will prevent acute attacks in susceptible persons. Thiazides may precipitate or aggravate diabetes.

Other diuretics. Spironolactone is as effective as a thiazide in the control of hypertension and is generally well tolerated but is

Table 13.2 Selected drugs suitable for routine management of hypertension. (For beta-blockers see Table 13.1)

Drug	Proprietary name	Dosage regime	Side effects
1. Diuretics			
Bendrofluazide	Centyl, Berkozide Aprinox, Neo-Naclex	2.5 to 5 mg daily	Hypokalemia Gout Diabetes
Spironolactone	Aldactone	50 to 200 mg daily	Hyperkalemia Gynecomastia
Indapamide[1]	Natrilix	2.5 mg daily	Nausea, Hyperuricemia
2. Vasodilators			
Hydralazine	Apresoline	25 to 100 mg twice daily	Headaches, flushing Systemic lupus erythematosus syndrome
Prazosin	Hypovase	0.5 to 20 mg, 2 to 3 divided doses (start with 0.5 mg nocte)	Postural hypotension (N.B. First dose effect – see text)
3. Others			
Methyldopa	Aldomet Dopamet	250 to 1000 mg thrice daily	Sedation, depression, impotence
Labetalol	Trandate	100 to 800 mg thrice daily	Postural hypotension (alpha-blockade) Bronchospasm, heart failure, lethargy (beta-blockade)

[1] Indapamide is not a diuretic at the dosage recommended

expensive. It may be used when a thiazide is contraindicated.

Indapamide, a recently introduced drug which has a direct effect on blood vessels similar to that of thiazides, but in the dosage given is not a diuretic, may be useful when hypokalemia is a problem.

Triamterene and amiloride have an inadequate effect on blood pressure when used alone but their potassium-sparing action makes them useful in combination with a thiazide in those prone to hypokalemia.

Frusemide should not be used routinely because it has less anti-hypertensive effect than thiazides. It may be useful, however, when heart or renal failure coexist with hypertension and a more powerful diuresis is required.

Beta-blockers

If control of blood pressure is inadequate on a thiazide alone, a beta-blocker is then added. All beta-blockers appear to lower blood pressure irrespective of whether or not they have cardioselective, membrane stabilizing or partial agonist properties. The mechanism of action is unclear. In general they are well tolerated and cause few unwanted effects. Postural hypotension and interference with sexual function are rare. In patients with angina they serve a dual function but should be used with caution under certain circumstances.

There is little to choose between the antihypertensive effect of the many products available (see Table 13.1). In the interest of patient compliance, once-daily medication is preferable to multiple doses. Hypertensive control is probably as good with once-daily medication with standard drugs as with the same dose of slow release formulation, although higher peak levels may produce more unwanted effects. Combined preparations containing beta-blocker and diuretic have the advantage of simplicity.

Beta-blockers may also be used satisfactorily in conjunction with vasodilators, alpha-blockers and other antihypertensives.

Vasodilators

If blood pressure remains inadequately controlled with a diuretic plus a beta-blocker, a vasodilator may be added.

Hydralazine has a direct effect on vascular smooth muscle causing vasodilation. It should not be used except in combination with a beta-blocker which prevents reflex sympathetic effects. Thus many of the side-effects, such as palpitations, headaches and flushing, can be minimized. Systemic lupus erythematosus syndrome may occur but is rare with doses of less than 200 mg daily.

Prazosin is now classified primarily as an alpha-blocker but it has some direct vasodilating properties. Unlike other alpha-blockers or vasodilators it does not tend to cause reflex tachycardia. Because it decreases cardiac work it may be of value in patients with heart failure who cannot tolerate beta-blockers. It has the disadvantage of causing postural hypotension and may produce a profound drop in blood pressure and collapse with the first dose, which does not occur subsequently. This may be prevented by starting with a small dose of 0.5 mg at night.

Other antihypertensives

Methyldopa is less satisfactory than beta-blockers but may be useful when a beta-blocker is contraindicated or poorly tolerated, or as an additional agent when control is inadequate. It acts mainly on central adrenergic pathways. It rarely causes postural hypotension but drowsiness and fatigue make it unsuitable for many patients, particularly the elderly and those whose work involves mental activity. Depression and impotence may occur. It may be useful in the management of hypertension in renal disease and pregnancy.

Labetalol is a promising new compound which has both alpha- and beta-blocking properties. It can be used to control hypertension of all degrees and it may be effective when other agents have failed. It may be used alone or in combination with a diuretic. Orally it works within two hours of starting therapy and maximum effect is achieved in four hours. It is generally well tolerated but may cause postural hypotension especially at higher doses.

Miscellaneous. Clonidine (Catapres), although an effective anti-hypertensive, may cause severe rebound hypertension if it is stopped suddenly, especially if the patient is also taking beta-blockers. It cannot, therefore, now be recommended for routine use.

Adrenergic neurone blockers, such as guanethidine, are used rarely because of postural hypotension and other side-effects but may be used in resistant hypertension.

Reserpine, once a popular drug, is now rarely used because it causes depression.

Can treatment be stopped?

In mild cases there is some evidence that about 15% of patients remain normotensive when treatment is stopped although the majority relapse, usually within nine months. In general, therapy is required for life, and this should always be made clear to the patient at the outset.

Hypertensive emergencies

The only indications for rapid lowering of blood pressure by the intravenous route are severe hypertensive left ventricular failure, dissecting aortic aneurysm, hypertensive encephalopathy and eclampsia. Intravenous diazoxide as a bolus of 75 to 100 mg is commonly used and acts within minutes. Intravenous sodium nitroprusside, labetalol and hydralazine are alternatives. Careful monitoring is essential as severe hypotension may be produced which can lead to a myocardial infarction, strokes and blindness from optic nerve damage. The present of accelerated hypertension by itself does not call for such drastic measures and can usually be managed by oral therapy, but hospital admission is usually necessary to ensure rapid control of blood pressure.

MANAGEMENT OF HEART FAILURE

Modern drugs have greatly improved the quality of life for many patients with heart failure. The failing heart is unable to expel its normal volume and thus dilates, increasing work and oxygen requirements. Rational therapy is directed towards reducing plasma volume with diuretics, increasing the heart's contractility by using positive inotropic agents and lessening pressure work with vasodilators.

The degree of severity of cardiac failure varies enormously, ranging from mild dyspnea on normal daily activity to severe dyspnea at rest in acute pulmonary edema. Urgency of treatment should be estimated at the start and therapy adjusted accordingly.

Underlying factors

Attention to underlying causes is important because specific therapy may be indicated, e.g. control of hypertension, antibiotics for infective endocarditis, or sodium retaining drugs, such as steroids. Heart rate is important. Insertion of a pacemaker in complete heart block or control of rapid atrial fibrillation with digoxin may lead to rapid resolution of heart failure.

General measures

Bed rest reduces energy requirements and alone will produce a diuresis and improvement of heart failure in about one-third of patients. If prolonged bed rest is needed oral anticoagulants are sometimes used because of increased risk of pulmonary embolism.

Diuretic therapy

Diuretics are the mainstay of therapy and should be continued, with increasing dosage if necessary, until the signs and symptoms of heart failure have improved and the patient is free of edema. Weighing the patient indicates when basal weight has been achieved. It may then be possible to reduce the dosage but in chronic cases it is rarely possible to stop diuretics altogether.

Thiazides

The general characteristics of the thiazide diuretics are discussed on page 200. Bendrofluazide taken in the morning is a suitable drug.

'Loop' diuretics

These powerful diuretics are usually reserved for patients who are resistant to thiazides or are in acute left ventricular failure. Frusemide is most popular. A single daily dose (from 40 mg up to 500 mg in severe cases) is usually given. An early evening dose may be advantageous as some patients find it interrupts their daily routine less and may prevent nocturnal breathlessness. Intravenous frusemide produces a rapid diuresis which is complete in four hours. Bumetanide has broadly similar properties.

Potassium loss

Marked potassium loss may occur in patients who have substantial diuresis and in those needing intensive diuretic therapy to remain free of edema. To prevent hypokalemia, increased dietary potassium (e.g. vegetables, bananas, fresh fruit juices) and potassium supplements may be given. Potassium chloride is available in slow release form (e.g. Slow K, 2 to 6 tablets daily) or as an effervescent tablet (e.g. Sando-K, 2 to 4 tablets daily). Combinations of a thiazide and potassium are available but the amount of potassium in these preparations is insufficient if hypokalemia is a problem.

Spironolactone, amiloride and triamterene are mild diuretics and have potassium retaining properties. They should be used in conjunction with a thiazide or 'loop' diuretic, assisting the diuresis and reducing potassium loss. It is important to monitor plasma potassium, as dangerous hyperkalemia can occur.

Inotropic agents

Digoxin

The routine long-term use of digoxin in congestive heart failure, long regarded as mandatory, is now being questioned. Although there is little doubt that digoxin has a positive inotropic action in the failing and non-failing heart when used acutely in sinus rhythm, sustained improvement has been difficult to demonstrate, provided the patient is on adequate diuretics. In contrast, in atrial fibrillation the important role of digoxin in the control of ventricular rate remains unchallenged. It should not be used routinely in those in sinus rhythm whose heart failure is adequately controlled on diuretics alone because of the hazards of toxicity, especially in the elderly and those with hypokalemia, but it is useful in those in sinus rhythm who are inadequately controlled by diuretics.

Unless there is urgency, a loading dose is unnecessary as a steady state digoxin level is reached in about a week. A daily dose of 0.25 to 0.5 mg will produce adequate blood levels in most patients; less may be needed where impaired renal function is present. Serum digoxin levels can be measured and may be helpful in adjusting dosage once a steady state has been reached. When more rapid digitalization is required a loading dose of 1 mg followed by 0.5 mg eight and 16 hours later, and then 0.5 mg daily, with subsequent adjustments according to response, is a well tried regime. Parenteral digoxin is not recommended. In long-term maintenance therapy a single daily dose is effective.

Other inotropic agents

Some new inotropic agents are being used in hospital practice for management of acute cardiac failure associated with low output. Dopamine and dobutamine are such compounds. They are related to noradrenaline and may effectively increase cardiac output without increasing heart rate and heart work. They are ineffective orally and are not suitable for long-term use.

Vasodilators

Vasodilator therapy appears to be an important advance in the treatment of severe heart failure that has responded inadequately to conventional therapy. Reducing the impedance to left ventricular output improves cardiac output, decreases heart volume and reduces venous pressure leading to improvement in symptoms. Initial observations were made using intravenous sodium nitroprusside but it has subsequently been shown that oral vasodilators, such as isosorbide dinitrate, hydralazine and prazosin have similar effects.

MANAGEMENT OF ACUTE PULMONARY EDEMA (see Table 13.3)

In an acute attack the patient will prefer sitting upright and, if available, oxygen in high concentration should be given to relieve hypoxia. Intravenous diamorphine or morphine relieves anxiety, depresses pulmonary reflexes reducing dyspnea, and dilates peripheral veins reducing venous return. Intravenous frusemide induces a rapid diuresis and removes edema from the lungs. Aminophylline given slowly intravenously over 5 to 10 minutes relieves bronchospasm and possibly improves renal blood flow and cardiac output. Oral digoxin may be given to control atrial fibrillation and to stimulate the failing myocardium. In severe cases which fail to respond the venous return may be reduced and cardiac output improved by venesection of 500 ml of blood: tourniquets applied to all four limbs, which are let down in rotation for 15 minutes in each hour, may serve a similar function. Positive pressure ventilation and vasodilators may be tried in hospital practice.

Table 13.3 Drugs used in the immediate management of pulmonary edema

Drug	Recommended dosage	Side-effects	Comments
Diamorphine (heroin)	5 mg i.v.	Vomiting, hypotension (less than with morphine), respiratory depression	Use antiemetic at same time e.g. prochlorperazine (Stemetil) 12.5 mg i.v. Caution in obstructive airways disease
Frusemide	20 to 40 mg i.v. slowly		Bumetanide (Burinex) 1 to 2 mg i.v. is an alternative
Aminophylline	250 mg i.v. slowly over 5 to 10 mins	Nausea, arrhythmias	Oxygenate the patient first if possible
Oxygen	40 to 60%	Respiratory depression in severe obstructive airways disease	Use 24% if in doubt
Digoxin		See Table 13.4 for details	

Table 13.4 Drugs used for the treatment of arrhythmias

| Drug | Adult dosage | | Side-effects and comments |
	Loading	Maintenance	
Digoxin (Lanoxin)	1 mg stat. 0.5 mg 8 hrly (3 doses) Avoid i.v.	0.0625 to 0.5 mg daily	Nausea, arrhythmias Caution in the elderly, hypokalemia, renal failure, Wolff–Parkinson–White syndrome Blood levels available
Beta-blockers 1. Propranolol (Inderal)	1 mg/min i.v. (maximum 10 mg)	10 to 160 mg thrice daily	Bronchospasm, heart failure, impaired response to hypoglycemia.
2. Practolol (Eraldin)	5 mg slowly i.v. (maximum 20 mg)	Not now available orally	May aggravate peripheral vascular insufficiency and conduction defects. Do not use with verapamil
Verapamil (Cordilox)	1 mg/min i.v. (maximum 10 mg)	40 to 120 mg thrice daily	Nausea, hypotension Avoid in heart failure Do not use with beta-blockers
Lignocaine (Xylocard)	1 mg/kg i.v. over 2 mins	2 to 4 mg/min i.v. infusion	Agitation, fits Lower doses needed in renal and liver failure

Drug			Comments
Quinidine (Kinidin, Kiditard)	—	500 to 1250 mg twice daily (slow release)	Nausea, cinchonism (tinnitus, dizziness, headache), hypersensitivity, ventricular arrhythmias. Use digoxin concomitantly in supraventricular tachycardias. Measure blood vessels
Disopyramide (Rythmodan, Norpace)	300 mg orally, 2 mg/kg i.v. (maximum 150 mg) over 5 mins	100 to 200 mg 6 hrly 0.4 mg/kg/hr by infusion	Anticholinergic. Caution in prostatic enlargement, heart block, heart failure
Procainamide (procainamide Durules, Pronestyl i.v.)	25 mg/min i.v. (total 1 g)	1 to 1.5 g thrice daily (Durules)	Hypotension, systemic lupus erythematosus syndrome. Avoid in heart block. Oral therapy – use only Durules. Measure blood levels
Mexiletine (Mexitil)	100 to 250 mg i.v. (25 mg/min) 4 mg/min 1 hr 400 mg stat. orally	2 mg/min i.v. 200 to 250 mg orally thrice daily 2 hrs after loading	Nausea, dizziness, visual disturbance, hypotension, bradycardias
Amiodarone	—	200 to 800 mg daily	Corneal microdeposits,? interferes with thyroid metabolism. Not yet generally available

N.B. i.v. drugs: all should be given under ECG control. Most are suitable for hospital use only

MANAGEMENT OF ARRHYTHMIAS

General principles of therapy

An electrocardiogram must be obtained to determine the nature of the arrhythmia. Ambulatory monitoring has facilitated precise diagnosis of transitory arrhythmias.

The type of treatment varies considerably according to type of arrhythmia and its effect on the patient. Healthy hearts tolerate faster rates for longer than those that are not. Knowledge of the patient's previous cardiac state is useful.

Underlying causes and precipitating factors should be sought. The past response of the patient to therapy may help in deciding the most appropriate course of action. The urgency of treatment will be influenced by symptoms and signs of cardiac decompensation which may follow an arrhythmia. Prophylaxis against further arrhythmias may be indicated. Measuring blood levels of anti-arrhythmic drugs may help achieve optimal therapeutic doses and prevent toxicity.

Commonly used antiarrhythmic drugs (see Table 13.4)

Digoxin

Digoxin slows conduction in the atrioventricular (AV) node and is, therefore, primarily of use in slowing ventricular rate in rapid supraventricular tachycardias, particularly atrial flutter and fibrillation.

Beta-blockers

The beta-adrenoceptor blocking activity of these drugs reduces the excitability of the myocardium and delays conduction in the AV node. This may slow the ventricular rate in supraventricular arrhythmias or terminate the arrhythmia altogether. Sinus tachycardia and atrial and ventricular extrasystoles may also be controlled by these drugs, and they may abolish palpitations associated with anxiety. They are not the first choice for treating acute ventricular arrhythmias and the evidence that they prevent sudden death in coronary heart disease is inconclusive.

Verapamil

Verapamil predominantly slows AV conduction. Intravenously it is very effective in terminating atrial tachyarrhythmias, especially those involving a re-entry circuit in the AV node. It may also be useful in slowing ventricular rate in atrial flutter and fibrillation. It does not seem useful in ventricular arrhythmias.

Lignocaine

Intravenous lignocaine is effective against many types of ventricular arrhythmia. In the coronary care unit, it is the usual initial choice for suppression of ventricular arrhythmias. It is not effective in atrial arrhythmias.

Quinidine

Quinidine is effective against both supraventricular and ventricular arrhythmias. It is used to maintain sinus rhythm after cardioversion of atrial fibrillation or flutter and may be used to suppress ventricular arrhythmias. Because of its side-effects, particularly ventricular fibrillation from toxic doses, it has been little used in recent years. However, modern sustained release preparations and monitoring of blood levels have improved safety. AV conduction is enhanced by quinidine, and in treating supraventricular tachycardias digoxin must be used concomitantly to prevent an increase in the ventricular rate.

Disopyramide

This drug is similar to quinidine but has fewer side-effects and it has, therefore, become popular in the management of acute and chronic atrial and ventricular arrhythmias. It is effective in the prophylaxis of arrhythmias after myocardial infarction and in reducing recurrence of arrhythmias after cardioversion.

Procainamide

Procainamide is effective in many arrhythmias but is not now popular because of its side-effects. It may suppress ventricular arrhythmias when other agents have failed. It is not suitable for long-term use because of the possibility of inducing a systemic lupus erythematosus syndrome.

Mexiletine

Mexiletine has similar antiarrhythmic properties to lignocaine and is active orally. It has produced satisfactory control of ventricular arrhythmias when used in the long term but its side-effects may limit its use.

Amiodarone

Amiodarone has been found to be useful in refractory arrhythmias especially paroxysmal atrial fibrillation. It may also suppress supraventricular and ventricular arrhythmias. It is not generally available at present.

Other measures to control arrhythmias

Cardioversion

Electrical cardioversion is frequently used in hospital for management of acute arrhythmias. It is indicated for ventricular fibrillation and tachycardia, and for supraventricular tachycardia when hemodynamic deterioration has occurred and other therapy has failed.

Pacing

Symptomatic bradycardias may need temporary or permanent pacing and age should be no bar to this valuable therapy. Tachyarrhythmias may sometimes be terminated by overdrive pacing.

Treatment of specific arrhythmias

Paroxysmal supraventricular tachycardia

Paroxysmal supraventricular tachycardia is usually due to a re-
entry circuit at the level of the AV junction and is common in otherwise healthy people. The tachycardia may be terminated by
vagotonic procedures, such as carotid sinus massage, the Valsalva
maneuver or swallowing a bolus of ice-cream, which all slow AV
conduction (see Figure 13.2). If this is unsuccessful and the patient
is not too distressed, bed rest and sedation may be all that is
required because in many patients the tachycardia terminates
spontaneously. If this does not occur, drugs which slow AV
conduction may be tried. Intravenous verapamil is the drug of
choice. Intravenous practolol is an effective alternative but
administration after verapamil must be avoided as marked bradycardia may ensue. Digoxin may be used but it takes longer to act.
When drug treatment is unsuccessful and urgency is required
electrical cardioversion is necessary. Occasionally it may be
possible to pin-point specific avoidable precipitating factors but
recurrent attacks may require prophylaxis with a beta-blocker or
oral verapamil.

Some patients have anomalous, fast conducting pathways which
are associated with a short PR interval on the electrocardiogram
(e.g. Wolff-Parkinson-White syndrome). Drugs decreasing the
conduction in these pathways (e.g. disopyramid, quinidine,
procainamide) may be effective in terminating supraventricular
tachycardias. However, digoxin is contraindicated because
conduction may be increased.

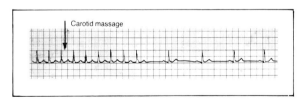

Figure 13.2 Paroxysmal supraventricular tachycardia terminated by carotid sinus
massage

Atrial fibrillation

The aim of therapy varies depending on the circumstances. In chronic atrial fibrillation, control of ventricular rate using digoxin is usually all that is required. If the ventricular rate on effort is excessive a beta-blocker may be added to provide control. When atrial fibrillation is of recent onset, particularly in younger patients and in those whose symptoms persist despite control of rate and underlying factors, cardioversion in hospital may be considered to restore sinus rhythm.

Atrial flutter

Control of rapid heart rates may be achieved by digoxin and/or a beta-blocker. Many of these patients will convert to atrial fibrillation. Underlying disease should be treated and cardioversion may be the treatment of choice, particularly when rapid control is needed.

Sinoatrial disease

This disorder tends to affect the elderly and may take the form of bradycardia alternating with tachycardia. It may prove difficult to treat. Pacing may be needed for the bradycardia and antiarrhythmic drugs to combat tachycardias.

Extrasystoles

Neither atrial nor isolated ventricular extrasystoles usually require therapy. Propranolol often controls troublesome symptoms: after myocardial infarction multifocal, frequent and early ventricular extrasystoles may require therapy.

Ventricular tachycardia

Acute attacks may be terminated by intravenous lignocaine (Figure 13.3). Alternatives such as disopyramide, mexiletine and procainamide may be tried. Electrical cardioversion is used in hospital when the patient has collapsed or has failed to respond to

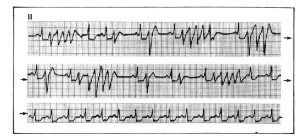

Figure 13.3 Paroxysmal ventricular tachycardia abolished by intravenous lignocaine (courtesy of Dr Andrew Mitchell)

drug therapy. Recurrent attacks may require long-term antiarrhythmic therapy.

Ventricular fibrillation

This is a common cause of death after acute myocardial infarction. A sharp blow over the praecordium with the fist may terminate the arrhythmia. If unsuccessful, external cardiac massage and ventilation are required until electrical cardioversion can be performed. Lignocaine may prevent a recurrence.

14
Future Prospects for the Treatment of Heart Disease

J. FLEMING

In the near future there is little prospect of achieving a break-through in our knowledge regarding the cause of our common heart diseases. While prevention remains the ultimate aim, we must continue with our efforts to increase the accuracy of diagnosis and refine the methods of treatment to minimize the effects of coronary atheroma, systemic hypertension, congenital heart disease, cardiac arrhythmias and heart failure.

SPECIALIZED CARDIAC INVESTIGATIONS

Angiocardiography

Modern angiocardiographic techniques provide a very detailed picture of the anatomy of the heart and show with great clarity any valve abnormalities or congenital defects. However, the procedure carries a risk to the patient because a catheter is inserted into the circulation, and a volume of radio-opaque contrast is injected that temporarily replaces the blood within the heart in its passage through the chambers which it outlines. Recent advances include technical refinements in the X-ray apparatus for the production of clearer pictures, such as the use of a caesium iodide screen and the development of radio-opaque contrast fluids of very low toxicity. But the total amount of contrast fluid that can be injected is still limited by the high osmolarity of these iodine-containing

219

compounds. New contrast fluids with low osmolarity and low viscosity are now available and are in clinical trial.

The basic objection to cardiac catheterization and angio-cardiography remains, that is, the risk involved in the introduction and manipulation of a catheter within the human body. This is an invasive technique and will eventually be replaced by new, non-invasive methods when these have been developed to the necessary degree of clarity and accuracy. Echocardiography and cardiac imaging using radioactive materials (radionuclide angiography) both offer some prospect of reducing our need for cardiac angiography.

Echocardiography

The first attempts at echocardiography provided a very limited picture of the heart. A single beam of sound was directed into the chest and the returning echoes from all the structures encountered in its passage through the heart provided a single dimensional 'ice-pick' view of the heart. Rapid to and fro movement of the beam or the use of a phased array of beams now allow a much larger area to be pictured. Sector scanning of the heart enables sectional moving pictures to be taken of the beating heart at many levels, both in the longitudinal and transverse planes. The anatomical information obtained is good and further developments will undoubtedly improve the clarity of the pictures. Echocardiography involves no risk and no discomfort for the patient but will probably not develop to the stage of superseding angiocardiography completely, since intracardiac pressures cannot be measured and the technique is limited to the examination of those parts of the heart that allow the echoscanner a pathway for its sound beams, free from intervening lung tissue.

Radionuclide angiography

Following the injection of a small volume of radioactive tracer into a peripheral arm vein, radionuclide angiography can now provide a picture of the heart chambers. Further developments in this technique will improve the frequency response of the recording equipment and provide more detail than is presently available.

Investigation of the heart's conducting system

A detailed study of the conducting system of the heart at present involves the insertion of many electrodes for stimulation and recording from the right atrium, bundle of His, right ventricle, left atrium and left ventricle, the results of which have greatly aided the diagnosis, mechanism and management of cardiac arrhythmias. From these detailed studies there should evolve a simplified scheme for the diagnosis and management of all but the most complicated cardiac arrhythmias. Already methods for recording bundle of His potentials from the surface electrocardiogram have been reported, and non-invasive methods for the determination of conduction pathways within the heart may well follow.

CARDIAC SURGERY

In coronary artery disease

Coronary artery bypass surgery is an established procedure for the relief of severe angina pectoris. The effect of this operation on long-term survival is not known, and a definite answer to this question is urgently required. The technique of the operation has reached considerable refinement and an operative mortality of less than 2% can now be achieved. Without surgery, multiple obstructions in the coronary arteries together with poor function of the left ventricle are known to be associated with a poor life expectancy, but it is also uncertain whether surgery improves life expectancy in these patients.

The precise place of coronary artery surgery in the treatment of coronary artery disease remains to be evaluated in the light of experience and further clinical trials. Present experience of coronary artery revascularization surgery in the first hours after myocardial infarction has generally been unfavourable. An acute obstruction in one or more coronary arteries is by no means always present at the onset of a myocardial infarction and the factors involved in the precipitation of infarction remain to be discovered.

In congenital heart disease

For congenital heart disease the surgical emphasis is moving away from palliation towards complete correction of the lesions. Transposition of the great vessels has hitherto been treated by the creation of an atrial septal defect in early infancy by using an inflatable balloon on the end of a cardiac catheter. Definitive cardiac surgery followed later when an intra-atrial baffle was inserted to divert blood from the right atrium to the right ventricle and aorta. This operation achieved considerable success but there were occasional complications with shrinkage of the baffle and arrhythmias, and the long-term prospects of the right ventricle maintaining a systemic blood pressure are not known. The emphasis in surgery at present seems to be moving towards the more radical procedure of reinsertion of the aorta and pulmonary artery into their appropriate ventricles. New surgical techniques enable this to be performed in infancy with a fairly low mortality.

Complete correction of Fallot's tetralogy is performed at present in infancy in selected favourable cases, and the continued progress in surgery for this condition makes it virtually certain that in the foreseeable future all cases will be treated in infancy in this way. Surgical reconstruction of severely deformed hearts is now possible using artificial conduits and homografts of aortic tissue. In the future surgery will be available for such conditions as truncus arteriosus and pulmonary atresia. Perhaps the only remaining problem in congenital heart disease will be the presence of severe irreversible disease of the pulmonary vasculature, the solution for which will require the emergence of a satisfactory operation for lung transplant.

Heart transplants

At present heart transplant operations offer the patient with severe myocardial disease the prospect of a few more years of active life.

Although this operation is once again available in England, this form of therapy may always be limited by the lack of suitable donor hearts. Efforts continue to develop a mechanical heart suitable for long-term implantation but as yet no promising design has emerged.

Cardiac pacemakers

Initially, an implanted cardiac pacemaker was used for the treatment of atrioventricular block accompanied by Stokes–Adams attacks. The indications for a permanent cardiac pacemaker have now broadened considerably to include the sick sinus syndrome, severe bradycardias of various etiologies and also some patients with paroxysmal tachycardia. Great progress in the design of pacemakers has resulted in miniaturization together with an extended battery life of 15 years or more.

The type most commonly used is the ventricular demand pacemaker which comes into operation to stimulate the right ventricle at a rate of 70 beats per minute whenever the ventricular rate falls below this level. In clinical practice its effect is usually satisfactory but the resultant heart contractions are far from ideal. More sophisticated pacemakers, which stimulate first the atria and, 0.2 seconds later, the ventricles, are now becoming available. Their action allows a regular sequential cardiac cycle of atrial contraction followed, after the appropriate time interval, by ventricular contraction.

Initial problems in the manufacture of an implantable unit have been overcome and it is now uncommon for a pacemaker to fail prematurely. Modern pacemakers are effectively screened from outside electrical interference and provided the patient is not exposed to high-energy electromagnetic radiation, such as by close proximity to a radio-transmitting aerial or to a malfunctioning micro-wave oven, are unlikely to be affected by extraneous influences. No damage results from a direct current shock because a special diode protects the electronic circuits from the possible ill effects of a transient surge of high-energy current. Short-wave diathermy does not harm the pacemaker but there is a possibility of myocardial damage from burning if the diathermy current becomes concentrated at the tip of the pacemaker electrode. Whenever possible, therefore, diathermy should be avoided in all pacemaker patients.

Pacemaker design

In all probability nuclear pacemakers will now be abandoned because of the many problems associated with using this type of energy source and its potential environmental hazards. Lithium iodide batteries with a projected life expectancy under normal load conditions of over 15 years have been developed, thereby removing the need to consider nuclear power. With this great advance in the power-source life, attention is once again turning to the design of long-lasting, stable pacemaker electrode wires. A flange near the tip of the electrode prevents most displacements but early and late movements of the electrode within the right ventricle cause a failure to pace in about 1% of all implants. Various ingenious electrode tips are under development, including the corkscrew electrode which screws into the myocardium, the 'christmas tree' electrode containing many tines just proximal to the tip, and the porous electrode whose tip becomes invaded by patient tissue within hours of being positioned in the myocardium. It is claimed that the rise in threshold to stimulation that occurs within the weeks after implantation is very much less in this porous electrode than with the more conventional electrodes. The wire must be pliable to avoid any danger of myocardial perforation yet very resistant to fracture. Usually the wire consists of several interwoven strands and the composite wire so formed is coiled in a tight spiral. Fractures do occur, however, and with the extended pacemaker battery life research continues to find the ideal wire that will reliably transmit pacemaker stimuli to the heart for 15 years or more.

'Programmable' cardiac pacemakers have now appeared that allow the rate and the duration of the pacemaker stimulus to be altered within wide limits at any time after implantation. A reduction of the pacemaker stimulus duration down to 0.1 or 0.2 msec offers considerable advantages as far as battery life is concerned, and can be attempted one month after implantation when no further rise in threshold to stimulation is to be expected.

The duration of the stimulus is reduced until it fails to capture the ventricle and a duration of twice this minimum value is chosen for long-term pacing. The ability to vary the pacemaker rate has not proved generally useful in clinical practice because the patient's physiological mechanisms usually allow him to vary his cardiac output quite widely according to his level of activity while the heart rate is held constant at 70 beats per minute. However, a few patients, usually those with severe impairment of myocardial function, are unable to alter ventricular stroke volume and can derive considerable benefit from a pacemaker whose rate can be programmed to suit the individual requirement. In children and for some forms of paroxysmal tachycardia a programmable pacemaker may well have a large role in the future.

Many forms of paroxysmal tachycardia are now recognized to arise on the basis of re-entry, the wave of electrical depolarization travelling continuously round an abnormal pathway in the heart. One or more small electrical stimuli will, if delivered at precisely the correct time, interrupt the circus movement of the tachycardia, and thereby restore sinus rhythm. Specialized pacemakers for permanent implantation, built to deliver small electrical stimuli when appropriately activated, are now under trial, and this method offers considerable hope for the future treatment of the paroxysmal tachycardias refractory to drug therapy.

CARDIAC DRUGS

Treatment of arrhythmias

From the first description of the use of digitalis in 1785, this drug has remained a mainstay of therapy despite the considerable problems regarding its toxicity and precise indications for use. In addition to its action in delaying the passage of impulses through the atrioventricular node, digitalis has vagal-stimulating properties and other complex effects on conduction velocity and in enhancing automaticity. For the treatment of some arrhythmias, particularly atrial flutter and atrial fibrillation, digitalis is the drug of choice, but for many abnormalities of cardiac rhythm new important drugs with rather more selective modes of action have been developed.

Thus amiodarone, a new drug which prolongs the refractory period of conducting tissue, is of great value in the treatment of the Wolff–Parkinson–White syndrome paroxysmal tachycardias, and verapamil, with its specific effects on conduction within the atrioventricular node, is very useful in the therapy of nodal tachycardia. But even these new drugs have unwanted side-effects, for example amiodarone causes corneal deposits and decreased myocardial contractility. Further new drugs will be developed with highly selective specific actions on the conducting tissues of the heart.

Treatment of heart failure

Many types of heart disease culminate in the production of signs and symptoms of heart failure. Efforts to stimulate the failing heart with digoxin usually meet with only limited success, and attention has been directed recently to reducing the work demanded from the heart. Resistance to forward flow of blood through the tissues of the body can be reduced by the administration of vasodilators, including prazosin, isosorbide dinitrate and hydralazine. These drugs can be quite effective in minimizing the effects of heart failure by reducing the 'after-load' on the heart. Hopefully, future vasodilators will be developed which have fewer of the unwanted side-effects of hypotension, tachycardia and the rapid decline in beneficial effects usually encountered with chronic administration of those presently available.

A mechanical method for reducing the heart's work-load is now available for short-term management of acute cardiac failure and consists of a large balloon connected to the end of a catheter. The catheter is inserted into the femoral artery through a surgical incision in the groin and the balloon is positioned in the descending thoracic aorta. Regular inflation and deflation of the balloon in sequence with the heart beat offers some degree of assistance to the failing heart, but because of the time limit on its use this balloon pump offers help in the management of an acute crisis rather than in long-term treatment.

Diuretics

Diuretic therapy remains the most direct line of approach for the relief of symptoms of heart failure because practically all these symptoms – dyspnea, abdominal distension and swelling of the legs – are caused by the retention of salt and water by the kidneys. The very potent oral diuretics now available, such as ethacrynic acid, frusemide and bumetanide, offer a very convenient means of forcing the kidneys to excrete sodium and water, but include amongst their undesirable effects an elevation of the serum uric acid and the possible aggravation of any tendency towards diabetes mellitus. A high serum uric acid level is obviously unfortunate in the patient with gout and in fact many patients suffer their first attacks of gout while taking diuretics for the treatment of heart failure. If a high serum uric acid carries other undesirable consequences for the future progression of coronary artery disease, then a uricosuric diuretic might be the drug of choice in the future. It has not been proven, however, that high serum uric acid alone predisposes to future cardiovascular disease.

Treatment of coronary artery disease

The search continues for a drug to prevent and to treat the build up of atheromatous plaques in the coronary arteries. Long-term anti-coagulants have been explored extensively in this context and found to be ineffective. On the hypothesis that platelet deposition may trigger off the pathological process, many trials are under way using antiplatelet drugs, aspirin, dipyridamole, and sulphinpyrazone, but results to date are not particularly encouraging.

A different approach is made by those who consider that the underlying defect is an abnormality of cholesterol handling within the body. Low cholesterol diets, clofibrate and cholestyramine are all used to lower serum cholesterol but the effect is minimal in established coronary artery disease. In fact, clofibrate can no longer be advised for routine use because of the increased incidence of gallstones and an adverse effect on mortality from non-cardiac causes in patients taking this drug. Progress in the drug therapy of coronary atheroma may well depend upon the development of an entirely fresh approach to the problem.

Index

229